Acclaim for Dan Shapiro's

Mom's Marijuana

"Part memoir, part social commentary, part medical journal and entirely wonderful."
—*Fort Worth Star-Telegram*

"We did not expect to laugh out loud over the story of a young man's battle with Hodgkin's disease. We also did not expect to finish it in one sitting, but there you have it—*Mom's Marijuana* is that terrific."
—*Arizona Republic*

"A wry, moving memoir of suffering and survival. . . . A paean to perseverance, a hymn to hope."
—*Kirkus Reviews*

"Affecting, witty and perceptive."   —*Publishers Weekly*

"The engaging and insightful tale of a healer whose practice is molded by his own experience of illness."
—*New Age*

Dan Shapiro

Mom's Marijuana

Dan Shapiro is an assistant professor in the department
of integrative medicine/psychiatry at the University of
Arizona Health Sciences Center. He lives in Tucson
with his wife, Teresa, and their two daughters.

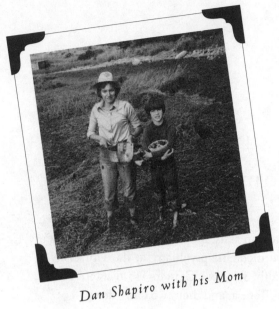

Dan Shapiro with his Mom

Vintage Books
A Division of Random House, Inc.
New York

Mom's Marijuana

Life, Love, & Beating the Odds

by Dan Shapiro

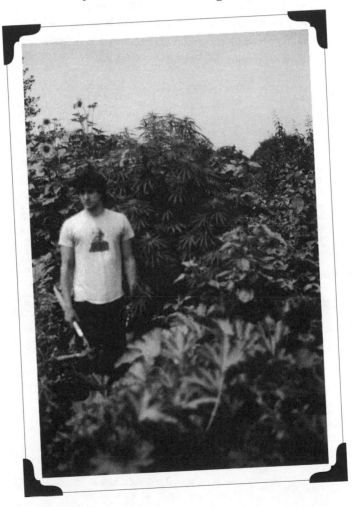

Author's Note: Any correlation between real life and events portrayed in this book is entirely intentional. With the exception of the names of most of my physicians, which I've changed, the rest is my perception. Any misinterpretation of reality found herein is due to quirky perspective, chemotherapy-induced memory loss, sleep deprivation, or all three.

FIRST VINTAGE BOOKS EDITION, SEPTEMBER 2001

Copyright © 2000 by Daniel E. Shapiro

The Library of Congress has cataloged
the Harmony edition as follows:
Shapiro, Dan
Mom's marijuana : insights about living / by Dan Shapiro.
1. Shapiro, Dan, 1966– 2. Physicians—Biography.
3. Marijuana—Miscellanea. I. Title.
R154.S3668 A3 2000
610'.92—dc21 00-38275
[B]

Vintage ISBN 0-375-70801-4

Book design by Christopher M. Zucker

www.vintagebooks.com

Printed in the United States of America
10 9 8 7 6 5 4 3 2 1

For T, little fish, and little blue,
you are my life's reward.

"I don't want to achieve immortality through my work;
I want to achieve immortality through not dying."

—WOODY ALLEN

Acknowledgments

I am in debt. Particularly to those who didn't make me change the title—even after a postal inspector ripped open two boxes carrying the book (on the off chance that I was smuggling mom's marijuana and had accurately labeled the boxes). I also owe Alan Gelenberg and Andy Weil, who were vigorous advocates at the University of Arizona.

I owe those who taught me to listen and appreciate: Andrew Arnold, Bruce Douglas and Frances Pass in Bloomfield, Connecticut. Karen Robertson, Janet Gray, Jim Steerman and Randy Cornelius at Vassar College, the best school in the country and where I learned to think and write. Stephen Boggs, Adam Fuller and Jeff Musick at the University of Florida. Arthur Klein, Bill Pollack, Joe Shay, Judy Jordan and Kate Mulrenin at McLean. And the best mentor a psychologist-in-training could have, Gerald Koocher, at Harvard Medical School, who taught me that there are many ways to be human and to be a psychologist.

I owe the many people who reached out to me at Vassar and the University of Florida, too numerous to list.

I owe some talented readers: Robby Lee, Donna Swaim, Ann Jones, Joann Munderloh, Angel Seibring, Mike Diesenhouse, Richard Liebowitz, Laura Basili, Lizzy Lauler, Andy Arnold, Andy Weil, Shauna Shapiro, Cindy Monheim, Russ Greenfield, Julia Greenfield and Ulrike Shapiro.

I owe Audrey Schulman, an author so accomplished that her books are sold even in truck stops, who took me aside on a snowy afternoon and taught me about details, commas, editors and agents.

I owe Amy Dickinson, a manuscript doctor and now a regular contributor at *Time,* who was willing to put my essays on N.P.R.'s *All Things Considered.* Without knowing it, she changed my life.

I owe a literary agent extraordinaire, Judith Riven, who heard one of my *All Things Considered* commentaries on her portable radio while walking in Central Park and was willing to shepherd me through the strange and wonderful business of publishing. Judith is a gift to any writer lucky enough to work with her.

I owe Jane Brody of *The New York Times* for her salmon recipe and generous journalism. I owe the amazing folks at Harmony, my editor and advocate, Shaye Areheart, and Tammie Ford.

I owe the book lovers of Vintage. Marty Asher, the meditating captain of the ship and his creative crew, Russell Perreault, David Hyde, Annsley Rosner, and my editor, Julie Doughty. I owe two dedicated readers who worked tirelessly with me to ensure that not a single word that didn't belong slipped into the manuscript. Jeff Musick, a man of great intelligence and character, and my brother, David Shapiro, whose creativity, laughter and honesty continue to inspire.

I owe my parents, Ann and Mark Shapiro, for everything.

I owe Teresa. More than I can speak.

Contents

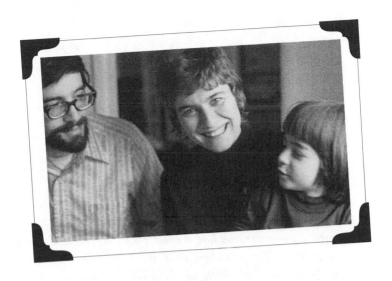

Part One

The Beginning

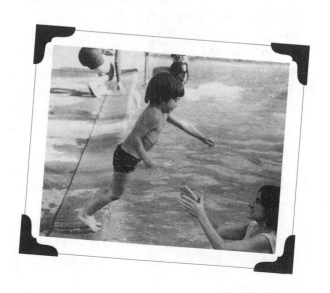

Dictated Chart Note

5/87

This is a 20-year-old white male who presented with a four week history of shortness of breath, wheezing, and night sweats. He was seen in an urgent care center and had a chest x-ray that revealed a large mediastinal mass. He was then seen at St. Francis Hospital in Hartford, Connecticut for further evaluation. At that time, a supraclavicular node biopsy was performed. Pathology findings of Reed-Sternberg cells in the specimen were consistent with a diagnosis of nodular sclerosing Hodgkin's disease. It should be noted that the patient reported a greater than 10 month history of classic B symptoms including fever, night sweats, chills, itching and nodal pain in right shoulder with the ingestion of alcohol.

Further CT evaluation of the patient revealed a >14 cm mediastinal mass and palpable supraclavicular nodes were noted bilaterally. There appeared to be no disease below the diaphragm. A bilateral bone marrow aspirate and biopsy revealed no bone marrow disease. Therefore, the diagnosis is Stage IIB nodular sclerosing Hodgkin's disease. Prognosis is good, the five year survival rate for Stage II Hodgkin's disease is 70%.

The patient will undergo six cycles of MOPP chemotherapy followed by mantle radiation. We anticipate that treatment will last approximately seven months.

CHARLES BRODSKY, M.D.
St. Francis Medical Center

Mom's Marijuana: Part A

My parents always kept a small plot of land in the backyard as a garden. It was roughly the size of an average bedroom. Pretty small. But they hovered around that garden all spring and summer. They plowed, fertilized, hoed, mulched, and sampled the soil. They watered. They pinched leaves. At night they pointed to pictures in books and seed magazines, which eventually accumulated and took over the dining room.

And then, a few months later, there was a crop of something. Usually a crop of mutant something. One year it was zucchini. Thousands of zucchini crawled out of the garden as if cast in a late-night horror film. Neighbors came home to anonymous zucchini breads, pies, and cakes delicately balanced inside of screen doors or stuffed into mailboxes. Dad kept a huge zucchini next to his bed in case there were intruders.

I was diagnosed with Hodgkin's disease in April, the planting month. Dr. Brodsky talked with his arms crossed in front of him, listing the chemotherapy agents I would be taking and their side effects. Prednisone. Procarbazine. Nitrogen mustard. Vincristine. The latter two would cause nausea and vomiting. It sounded unpleasant.

A few nights before I was scheduled to start treatment, I called a friend, the only person my age I knew who'd had cancer. He muttered five gruff words into the phone: "Chemo's grim, man, get weed."

I trotted into the living room and nonchalantly announced to the family that I was going to buy marijuana to help with the nausea and vomiting.

There was an oppressive silence, punctuated only by the rapid tapping of my mother's finger on an armchair. Then she began, her voice carrying that staccato edge she generally reserved for my father. She told me in no uncertain terms that there would be no drugs in the house. She berated me about the dangers of illicit substances, the horrors that visit lives filled with addiction, and swore to me that her roof would never shelter a drug user. She ended her diatribe with an outstretched finger.

With the vigor of an adolescent with a cause, I argued back that for me, marijuana would be medicine, the only medicine that could temper the violent treatment I faced. That it wasn't addictive, and that my body would soon process toxins far more dangerous than marijuana. At the end of our conversation we were where we began. I knew my mother. Once she was entrenched in a position, argument was futile. I retreated.

I still wonder what happened to her during the night. Maybe she studied the pamphlets the doctors provided, maybe she woke up in a sweat, the remnants of noxious dreams about her son and chemotherapy still etched in her mind's eye. I don't know. But I do know this. The next morning my mother ran her finger down the "Smoke Shop" listings in the phone book. She called a number of establishments, asking detailed questions and jotting down words like *bong, carb*, and *water pipe*. Then she gathered her keys and purse, and thirty minutes later was walking down the aisles of a head shop called Stairway to Heaven, taking notes and carefully checking the merchandise for shoddy workmanship. My mother is a *Consumer Reports* shopper.

I was sitting on the ground in the backyard when my mother's car pulled into the driveway. A few moments later she appeared on the back porch waving a three-foot bong over her head. She proclaimed her find with the same robust voice she'd used for years to call my brother and me to dinner: "Is this one okay? They didn't have blue. . . ."

When I entered the house she delicately handed me the bong and some money. She brushed dust from my shoulder and softly told me to do whatever I needed to get the marijuana. After a quick phone call I left to make my purchase. When I returned with the small Baggie my mother asked to see it. I felt a sharp adolescent fear, conditioned from years of living under my mother's vigilant eyes. I handed it over. She looked into the small bag. Incredulous.

"Where's the rest of it?" she asked.

"That's it, Ma," I said. She squinted at me. "I swear, Ma. That's it."

She murmured quietly, "Honey, give me the seeds."

I thought of huge zucchinis.

When my father learned of my mother's plan he clipped two articles out of the paper with the titles "Police Raid Yields Results" and "Drug House Seized." He put them under a magnet on the refrigerator and underlined the worst parts. That night, as we prepared for dinner, Mom read them, nodded soberly, and said, "Bring them on."

That summer my parents plowed, fertilized, hoed, mulched, and sampled the soil. They watered. They pinched leaves. And that August the mutant crop arrived. Ten bushy plants grew over eleven feet tall in our backyard, eclipsing the sunflowers in front of them. Far more weed than I could have smoked in a lifetime.

Pretzels

When I was thirteen I stashed three issues of *Penthouse* between my mattress and the box spring. My mother found them during a cleaning tirade and angrily marched them to the trash bins. Some of what she said was muffled, but I did hear the words *objectification*, *gynecological*, and *disgusting*. When she came back in, I told her the magazines were mine and she had no right to go in my room or throw my stuff out. I went and fished them out of the trash. We ended up facing each other, silent, outside my room. As we stood there I noticed that I'd tucked the magazines under my arm like a favorite blanket. I began to feel awkward and embarrassed. *Is this a battle I want to wage?*

I was about to hand them over when Mom's face softened. She nodded and whispered, "You know what? It's okay. I can think of worse things for you to be doing. You keep them." She spun on her heels and walked away.

We never talked about my sexuality again.

The tumor was fourteen centimeters wide. A grapefruit. There weren't many things it could be other than cancer. After the biopsy I had a host of tests to identify its species and preferred habitat. I reclined on tables under hovering machines, breathed into long purple tubes and allowed polite attendants to tap veins and arteries. Blood gases were drawn, lung volume was measured, and bone was aspirated.

Over those first weeks we learned that more time would be spent waiting for tests, and talking with Dr. Brodsky about results, than actually having the tests themselves. My mother accompanied me to the more difficult procedures, armed with a paperback or a crossword puzzle. She frequently started conversations with other patients or family members.

On one particular day we sat waiting for a bone marrow aspiration. I was pretending not to be nervous. I'd heard the procedure involved bone and needles. These were two words that, in my humble opinion, had no business appearing in the same sentence. I flipped through a *New Yorker*, trying to stay occupied. One other woman waited in the room. She was my mother's age, late forties or early fifties. She looked tired and gazed at nothing in particular, her face patient and stoic, her purse balanced on her lap.

After a while my mother looked up, smiled at her, and she smiled back. The woman's face warmed and then they were talking. Her son was having a spinal tap, a procedure where they take a small amount of fluid from the spinal cord. He didn't want her in the room during the procedure. "He's fourteen; he doesn't want me to see him cry," she explained. My mom nodded and tilted her head toward me as if to say, "They're all the same." Mom asked about her son's illness and the woman described his form of leukemia, expertly listing the chemotherapy drugs he'd taken and the amount of radiation. My mother told our short story. How they'd found the tumor and that Dr. Brodsky was trying to learn how far the disease had traveled from its first home in my chest. The woman smiled and nodded sadly, as if she were a veteran returning from the front meeting fresh-faced reinforcements.

Then they talked about side effects. Her son was halfway through treatment. He'd had nausea. Fatigue. Moodiness. He was probably sterile now. Mom asked questions. What had they tried to ease the harsher side effects? What had worked? What hadn't? How was his school handling his absences? Then the woman's expression changed. Her eyes opened a little wider and she leaned toward my mother. "Has he banked sperm?" she asked, nodding in my direction.

I looked up.

"Sperm?" asked my mother, loud enough for folks in distant zip codes to hear.

"He should bank sperm. I had my son do it," she encouraged.

"I didn't realize the treatment would make him sterile, the doctors haven't said anything," Mom responded, talking faster than usual.

"The doctors won't tell you about it, but you should do it. There's a doctor, a urologist in town, who has a sperm bank.

Wait . . ." She fumbled in her purse. "Ah, here it is!" She produced the number from a small book and wrote it on an envelope.
She smiled and handed it across the small room.

Then they both looked at me.

When Dr. Brodsky called me back for the aspiration my mother
tapped him on the arm and said she had something to discuss.
She explained that she wanted to wait to start treatment so we
could explore donating sperm. She made it sound as if we were
giving something very important to a charitable organization.

Dr. Brodsky wanted to start chemotherapy immediately. The
tumor was wrapped around my trachea. He told us there wasn't
much time to spare. I thought he was exaggerating but also
enjoyed the drama — I felt special, like a martyred hero in a World
War II movie.

I felt like saying, "Don't worry, General Patton, I'll hold on."
The truth was, since the diagnosis, I felt better. For the last year I'd
been having some odd symptoms but never connected them. I'd
had night sweats, dizzy spells, and intense pain in my shoulder
when I drank alcohol. It was satisfying to know what was wrong
and have a plan of attack. I was also getting twelve hours of sleep a
night, watching movies, and friends were visiting. If it weren't for
the strange way everyone asked how I was, necks craned forward
in sympathy, I wouldn't know I was sick. I was in no rush to start
chemotherapy.

"Wait here," he told us and left the room. He came back a few
moments later with one of my CAT scans. He put it up in the
view box. It was a cross section of my chest, a black-and-white
photograph of my insides as if I'd been sawed in half.

He cleared his throat, looked at my mother, and pointed with
a pen to a pea-sized hole surrounded by a hostile black acre of
tumor. "That's his windpipe. It should be the size of a quarter.
That's why he can't breathe well."

I studied the map of my internal geography. I touched the pea-sized hole with my finger. It was white. When I inhaled I heard and felt the raspy wheeze of air flowing through a very small space.

An electric pulse of reality thumped through my chest. I felt the world slow to a crawl. I heard the hum of the air conditioner and the fluorescent lights. I noticed the way Dr. Brodsky cleared his throat and involuntarily sighed between sentences. I felt the crinkle paper beneath me and could smell lingering cologne from some prior patient now gone. And then the weight. The sheer heaviness that pinned me to the spot as if my life had paused.

While I dissociated, silent and drifting, my mother and Dr. Brodsky settled on ten days.

Over dinner my parents discussed details. My mother had called the urologist's laboratory. It would cost only a few hundred dollars per year for storage for as long as we wanted. There was some evidence that sperm could last up to ten years, maybe longer. They'd put it in vials and store it in liquid nitrogen. When it was thawed, someday, most of it would still be alive.

The other details were a little unsettling. The laboratory was across town and it didn't have a patient waiting area. The lab technician emphasized the need for the "donation" to get to the laboratory within thirty minutes of exiting my body. This meant I'd have to do my part at home and then my parents would make the delivery.

My father disappeared into his study and came back with automobile club maps of Hartford and Bloomfield. He carried a pencil, pad, and calculator. As I cleared the dishes, my father spread the maps out on the table. He wrote down the rush-hour times and the speed limit on the thoroughfares. He highlighted the best route. He talked about "traffic density" and "stoplight-to-distance ratio." When I was done with the dishes I sat down between my parents.

My mother had one of her little notebooks open and was chewing on a pen, her feet up on a chair. My brother, David, had retreated into his bedroom after dinner. It wasn't his turn to do the dishes. He wandered into the kitchen in time to hear my mother say, "Okay, at ten you masturbate, then me and Dad will drive your sperm in. Then we're going shopping—anything you want from the grocery?"

"Uh, I guess, yeah, Ma, get me some pretzels," I said.

She wrote my request in her notebook.

We all looked up at David. "Anything you want, honey?" she asked him.

He squinted at all of us. Scratched his neck. Turned. Walked slowly back to his bedroom.

On the morning of the first deposit my mother stood outside my old bedroom door. In front of the house the car was running, my father perched like Mario Andretti behind the wheel of the eight-year-old Chevy Citation. I sat on my old bed, surrounded by the trappings of my adolescence: a poster of Blondie, bright orange drapes, a rusting trumpet, and a varsity wrestling letter pinned to the wall. I bent over the bed and found the magazines with my fingers, working them out from under the mattress, first forward, then back, like always.

I heard my mother shift her weight outside my door. I flipped through one of the magazines and tried to concentrate. If ever there was a time for a tour of the pornography hall of fame, this was it. For a while I was distracted by logistics. I couldn't decide how to hold the donation cup and the magazine and still have a free hand. Then I noticed I could hear the Chevy from inside my room. *When is Dad going to get that damned muffler fixed?*

Eventually familiar photographs of soft curves, skimpy under-wear, and long hair propelled the process along. It culminated in the strange and delicate job of getting as much of the magical sub-stance as possible into the container while my eyes rolled and feet quivered. In hastily pulled-up sweatpants I raced to the door and gave Mom the cup. She was all business.

"Pretzels, right?"

"Yeah, Ma. Pretzels."

She bounded out to the car.

Mom's Marijuana: Part B

My first exposure to marijuana came when I was in sixth grade. It occurred on the late bus. There were four late buses to serve the middle school and junior high. Any kid who stayed after school for detentions or sports, or, in my case, for band practice, had to take one of the late buses home. The late bus was always packed and took forever to get to my neighborhood. Donald, who'd moved from Jamaica two years before, drove my late bus. He was tall, thin, and had shiny black skin. I liked to listen to his accent and the funny things he said so I sat up front. Sometimes he'd sing, sometimes he'd tell us stories about Jamaica, and other times he'd make fun of us.

On this day, like every other day, I lugged my trumpet case up the steps and sat down a few seats from the front. The bus was even more crowded than usual. As Donald pulled out of the park-ing lot I could tell there was something different about him. He was quiet and he kept glancing up into the mirror directed back at all of us. He drummed one fist on the steering wheel and his eyebrows were tightly lowered. I thought he might be angry because the bus was so crowded and it was going to take him a long time to get back to his wife. "She got a body that live in your head, ya know," he'd said once, tapping a finger on his temple.

I turned and looked back into the bus. There were kids twisted around in their seats, throwing things, and a few smoked but this wasn't unusual. Most of the kids had been serving detentions for swearing, fighting, or smoking on campus. Many of them smoked and Donald had warned them not to burn the seats. It seemed an unwritten code that smoking was okay. I turned back around and stared out the window at the dry patches of snow in front yards and on rooftops.

Then, suddenly, Donald abruptly pulled the bus over and stopped. We were on Blue Hills Avenue, a busy road. I slid across the seat and into the kid sitting next to me. Donald was up quickly, his frame filled the walkway, and he bounded to the back of the bus. His deep baritone voice carried: "Ya risk my job when you smoke the cigarette. Ya risk my life when you smoke the ganja!" He reached a powerful arm into a cluster of kids sitting three in a seat, plucked one out and violently dragged him the length of the bus by his collar. At the front he kicked a few times at the door release and then pulled the kid down the stairs. I watched him gently push the kid onto the sidewalk and then a moment later Donald was back on the bus, the door was closed, and we were pulling away. I watched the kid on the sidewalk. His blond hair was rumpled and I could see his black T-shirt, partially untucked, hanging out under a denim jacket. His mouth was open and he looked bewildered, as if he'd just awoken to find himself in a strange country.

My second exposure to marijuana was on a wrestling mat. It was during hell week, the first week of practice. I was wrestling Eugene, a stocky kid who had a big mouth. I'd already wrestled one season and was virtually guaranteed a varsity spot. Eugene was trying out for the first time. I'd always been scared of him and didn't want to wrestle him. He fought a lot, argued back with teachers, and walked with a "pimp," bobbing and weaving down the hallways. When I stared at him in homeroom once, after he'd just yelled at a teacher, he barked at me, "What the fuck are you looking at?" and I'd looked away, voiceless.

Coach paired us up and I threw him down as quickly as I could, scared. I ran a chicken wing and pinned him quickly. "Fucker," he grunted. We set up again and I used a sun-devil, trapping his foot, and then a half nelson, pinning him again. Then I got fancy, using a bow and arrow to wrap him up tightly in a ball so his face would press uncomfortably against his knee. Coach Douglas blew the whistle and quietly said, "Stand up." We stood. Coach walked up to Eugene and me, putting his face close to Eugene's. "Eugene, you're slow as mo-las-ses. You been smoking the mar-i-ju-an-a?"

Eugene considered his answer. "Yeah, Coach." And he smiled with honesty.

Coach smiled back at him. "You're cut. There's the door."

At Vassar I found a different prevailing opinion of marijuana. Unlike in high school where marijuana smoking seemed as exotic and dangerous as opium, at Vassar (like most colleges in the mid-eighties) most students felt that marijuana was benign. Fellow students assumed that smoking marijuana shouldn't interrupt ambitions or studying. It was considered a less disruptive way of relaxing than keg parties. I'd only been there one week when a group of juniors gathered the freshmen of Joss dorm together and taught us marijuana etiquette, like always offer the first hit to one's guests and never throw out a joint remnant without first offering it to him or her.

Of students who used marijuana, most smoked only once a month or so. There was one heavy user on my hall. He smoked all day, even when he first woke up. We called him Wake & Bake. I remember shuffling down the hallway in my shorts toward the showers, a towel in one hand and shampoo in the other, hearing the sound of air being drawn through water, rapid bubbling, and then silence. This was followed by a strong exhale, a few coughs, and then the pungent smell wafted into the hallway.

"Mornin', Wake & Bake!" I'd yell.

A gritty "Yo" would respond. Wake & Bake could go to classes stoned. He even got good grades. I think he works at the Pentagon now.

I didn't smoke during the first few months of college. It wasn't offered and I wasn't interested. The first time I smoked was with Gokhon, a worldly Turkish student who was very bright and had traveled all over the globe. We'd studied together for an art history exam, memorizing more than three hundred slides of various artifacts. Paintings. Sculptures. Ceilings. Stairs. Monuments. Churches. We knew about mosaics and triptychs, oils and watercolors. Right after the exam Gokhon borrowed a car and told me to meet him in his room after dinner. He returned with a contraption of wood, glass, and rubber tubing. It was in the shape of an hourglass and the tubes ran this way and that. It was my first exposure to a bong and I thought it looked mysterious and scientific. Gokhon put a nip of the herb in a small bowl, lit it, and handed me the tube. I inhaled. Smoke swirled inside the glass and bubbled through water at the base. At first I didn't feel anything. Then I felt my body lift out of the chair, my limbs light and airy, and the room began to tilt. The smoke danced toward the ceiling and Gokhon smiled and patted my shoulder in friendship. I laughed and then he was laughing and soon we were afloat, utterly stoned. Thoughts came and went, too fast to discuss. Gokhon started talking about a painting we'd memorized—he'd actually seen it in Florence—but I couldn't pay attention. I was busy watching the black hairs on his head peeking up through the yarn of his beret, like frozen blades of grass peeking through dry snow.

We smoked about once a month our freshman year, usually on weekend nights and when we had access to food. Gokhon and I learned quickly that it was delightful to eat when we were high but also that we had to pace our eating. Messages from our stomachs to our brains were severed, and we could eat prodigious quantities of pizza, popcorn and other textured treats far beyond our stomach's capacities. If we weren't careful we'd awaken the next morning bloated and sluggish. We invented rules. For example, we allowed ourselves only one large Napoli's pizza between us per night and we avoided foods requiring much secretion to swallow. We noticed that our mouths were dry when we smoked; a mouthful of peanut butter could take a few seasons to ingest.

We also learned that if we smoked slowly and titrated our intake we could reach a place where we could think relatively clearly and enjoy intense and insightful conversations, as if our perspective on reality was angled, but not totally distorted as with alcohol. Too much weed, though, and we were unable to concentrate, let alone communicate. And worse, the days following were filled with apathy and word-finding problems.

Smoking to counter the effects of chemotherapy was different. All of my chemotherapy "hits" were scheduled in the morning. On those days I always awoke too early. Even in the twilight between wakefulness and sleep, when colors and adventure merge with alarm clocks, even then I knew. *It's a chemotherapy day.* After quickly dressing I would sit down to prepare the marijuana. It wasn't like with Gokhon, playful or exploring. It was business. Vocational.

The bong my mother provided was roughly the diameter of a sink pipe, with a wider bulb at the bottom. A small bowl, like on a traditional pipe, was attached to a small tube that descended into the wider bulb. I filled the bulb with water and ice. Then I cleaned the weed, separating twigs and seeds from the sticky green clumps of leaves. When I had a thimble full of clean weed, I delicately placed a pinch in the bowl. Now it was ready.

After my first chemotherapy hit, I didn't smoke. I had to see for myself that the chemotherapy would make me sick. Consequently, I spent the afternoon and most of the night making rapid trips to the bathroom to release the contents of my stomach. Before finally settling off to sleep, I asked Mom when she expected her crop to come in. "Depends," she said. "I don't think the *Farmer's Almanac* lists this particular crop. My guess is July or August. Maybe next time you should try to use the stuff you bought?"

During the second treatment I experimented with Marinol, the synthetic version of marijuana. Dr. Brodsky said he wasn't comfortable with me smoking marijuana without first trying a pill form of the drug. I'd learn later that Marinol is almost completely THC, just one of the many active ingredients in marijuana. Forty minutes after I took the white pill I was more stoned than I'd ever been with Gokhon. It was an unrelenting chemical high, the difference between one shot of vodka and twelve. I lost my balance. I couldn't put together a sentence. I lay prone in my bed, unable to move, trapped with a wandering consciousness. I didn't like it.

From then on I smoked marijuana. I smoked a little before leaving the house. My research in Vassar's library suggested that as many as 40 percent of patients getting chemotherapy got sick even before the chemo infusions because, like Pavlov's dogs, they were conditioned. It made sense to me to smoke a tiny bit before going, trying to reach that same place where Gokhon and I traveled most comfortably.

My father frequently had the task of driving me to chemo-therapy treatments. This led to some interesting conversations. We'd be driving to the hospital and I'd break the silence with, "How come everyone who believes in reincarnation thinks they were someone really important in a prior incarnation, like Napoleon or Cleopatra? No one ever says, 'I think I was the village idiot.'" Having no experience with marijuana himself, at least that he would admit, my father was perplexed. He knew I wasn't dangerous but didn't understand the sudden turns of my attention or why I had difficulty following a train of thought. Then I'd invariably ask, "We don't have any food in the car, do we?" Before he could answer I'd be off on another tangent. "Have you ever looked at your fingers? I mean *really* looked at them?"

When we arrived at the hospital I checked in and sat in the small waiting room with the other patients. Then Faye or one of the other nurses would call me back. Before I could get chemotherapy, she checked my blood counts by withdrawing a few cc's of blood and sending them to the lab. If my white blood count went too low, the chemotherapy would leave me vulnerable to life-threatening infections. This process reminded me of checking to see whether a convict on death row was healthy enough to be executed, but I never shared this observation with Faye.

I waited after the draw, and then Faye would reappear. By now the weed's effect had diminished and I was nervous. Faye liked to offer her arm as if she were ushering me to get an award and we'd walk back to a long room with a row of green recliners covered with plastic. Most of the chairs were occupied with folks sleeping or watching television, their arms hooked up to long plastic hoses. Some were behind curtains, where there were whispers, low talking, and the ever-present sound of the television.

In the world of chemotherapy cocktails, my mix was particularly noxious. Nitrogen mustard. Vincristine. Procarbazine.

High-dose prednisone. I was secretly proud to be getting the hard stuff and doing relatively well. Of the group, nitrogen mustard had the most notorious lineage. Brodsky told me that doctors had discovered it had the potential for helping in Hodgkin's disease when an explosion of nitrogen mustard gas in Naples harbor during World War II resulted in seamen having lymph gland responses. The drug caused considerable nausea and thinned hair. The other drugs were no kinder. Vincristine caused a bit more nausea and vomiting but was more infamous for its neurological side effects like numbing of fingers and toes. Procarbazine, an MAOI (monoamine oxidase inhibitor) similar to the antidepressant phenelzine, fiddled with neurotransmitters and caused mood swings. High-dose prednisone also altered mood and interfered with sleep. Generally, once the infusions started, I had forty minutes to get to the marijuana before the nausea and vomiting started. I could feel it building, like floodwaters pressing against a levee of sandbags. As soon as the infusions were over, Dad and I hustled out to the car. We kept buckets in the backseat just in case, but I only needed them once or twice. We considered having me smoke in the car, but concerns about police prevented this.

Dad drove with concentration and I rested my head against the side window, counting the stoplights until relief. Once home I quickly went into the house and down to my room. The first pull of smoke through the bong was liberating. Soon after I inhaled I felt relaxation soothe the back of my neck, shoulders, and stomach. As I exhaled I could watch the smoke turn and ascend and feel the violence disappear, my insides change from heavy downpour to light drizzle, raging white water settle to glass.

Waiting Rooms

I was diagnosed when I was completing my junior year at Vassar. I drove home to Bloomfield from Poughkeepsie twice a month to get chemotherapy. Unlike Vassar, a culture of mostly white late adolescents and young adults, the chemotherapy waiting room was populated with young and old; black, white, and Hispanic.

Once I sat next to an older, heavyset African-American woman in a wheelchair. She wore an elaborate plaid scarf on her head and crescent moon earrings. She smelled of sage and peppermint. We both had puffy features and circles under our eyes. As we were waiting our turns, we began to chat. She was knitting a sweater. It was ornate, a pattern of diamonds, violet and gold. Yarn bounced on her lap and her thick hands darted here and there, the needles prancing and pausing, prancing and pausing. I'd covered my bald head with a round and colorful beanie that sported a plastic propeller. She remarked about the beanie and I asked her who the sweater was for. She leaned forward and whispered.

"Every time I get a new doctor, I tell him I'm gonna knit him the most amazing sweater ever touched by human hands. The softest, warmest garment, he won't ever want to take it off. People for miles will come to see it. He'll want to sleep in it, eat in it, visit family in it, tend to patients in it, go to church in it, ride the bus in it"—and she got louder, her voice a deep church-nurtured baritone—"bathe in it, sing in it, swim in it. Then, and here's the important part . . ."

She paused for effect. Looked around as if we might be overheard.

"I never quite finish it." She stopped again. Leaned even closer. Raised a finger in the air.

"And you know what?" she asked. I shook my head no. Eyebrows raised. She winked at me. "They always keep me alive!" She threw back her head, erupted with an infectious cackle and the room was filled with our giggling.

Edi

My mother says she knew he'd died before anyone told her. She said she felt it. Even before the teacher crouched in front of her and held her hands. Soon after there was a somber funeral. And then she helped her brother and mother pack for America.

When he finally relaxed, his daughter, son, and wife were safe. There was no more Gestapo. No more air-raid sirens. No more internment camps. No more whistling incendiaries dropped from high above. And no more long hours in the munitions factory. Having barely escaped Austria and the Nazis, he died, probably of tuberculosis, in the Lake District of Northern England, when my mother was eight.

There were magical stories about him behind every creased black-and-white photograph in Nana's dusty albums. When I was young, Nana, my grandmother, called him Edward with a formality I didn't understand, her stories speckled with German and Yiddish. Over the years she softened and called him Edi. When we were alone she told me stories about him.

"He could fix anyzing," she told me. "Vonce he picked his vay into a safe to retrieve ze keys ze safe owner had left inzide." And "Vonce he built a bomb shelter under ze stairs by breaking down valls and hammering together pieces of vood he found on ze street. It zaved our lives when the bombs came."

On another visit she told me about his generosity. "The winter of 1940 was cold for us. Zey dropped bombs, ve had no heat. You know vat he did? In ze middle of a vinter rainstorm Edi gave his coat to a poor English woman. She vas cold, you understand?"

"'Ilse, ve owe zis country our lives,'" he told Nana when she protested.

And he worked harder than anyone she'd ever known. "All ze time, he worked. And never complained." Any work he could get. He was handy and capable. He could design something and build it.

Nana grew up in an affluent family. She was the younger of two daughters born to the owner of a shoe factory in Vienna. There were maids and dances and long dresses, operas and literature. On a hot summer night in Vienna he asked her to dance. She was pretty. There were plenty of other boys, but they were stiff and somber inside their vests. He wasn't well dressed, but he was gaunt like a romantic hero and he made her laugh. He was tall and moved easily as if he were going somewhere important. And when he spoke his face smiled and she found herself smiling. After a brief romance they were married. As she learned more she realized that his gaunt cheeks were the product of years of undernourishment. He also had a sister sick with epilepsy. He had to work to support her and his mother. When he was seventeen, he'd had his first case of tuberculosis, the European poor man's disease. Nana's father was not excited about the union. But she would not be swayed.

When I visited her, I'd dig through her closets looking for hints of him. They were there—an old cap that never moved, a tattered scarf. She kept his picture on her nightstand, a black-and-white photograph penciled in to give it color. In it his face is thin, but his cheeks are as bright as bougainvillea leaves. He looks beyond the camera with eyes that look like they have seen too much.

More than the reminders of his absence, it was Nana's resolute answer to a single question that conveyed the power of his presence in her life. I was eleven or so, curious and hyper, wrapping myself high around the willow tree in our backyard while she knitted below. I called down to her.

"Nana, how come you never remarried?"

There was no answer for a time and I surveyed a branch. Grabbed it, found another. Still nothing. I waited.

"I am married," she said quietly.

Eight months before I was diagnosed with Hodgkin's disease, when I was nineteen years old and the first symptoms, unknown to me, were emerging, I went looking for Edward. I wanted to find his grave. Before I left I sat down with Nana and asked her everything she remembered. She described the town where he was buried, gave me a pencil drawing of the cottage they were living in when he died in Northern England, and told me again how they, two Austrian Jews, happened to be there.

Vienna in the 1930s was unsafe for Jews. Austria's government had resisted National Socialism for over ten years. There were riots in 1927 and arguments on street corners, in barbershops, and in the Parliament. Nana and her family ignored them. But eventually the mostly Catholic country aligned behind the Pan-German party, which held that Austria and Germany should be reunited. German troops marched into Vienna, welcomed by most Austrians, in March of 1938. The Nuremberg Laws, established three years earlier in Germany, suddenly applied to Austrian Jews. The most important of the Nuremberg Laws for my family covered occupations. Jews were forbidden from holding professional jobs. Edi lost his job as an engineer, a job he'd starved through college to get. Unbroken, he sold shoes, did carpentry, and repaired engines. He got permission from the Gestapo to organize classes for displaced Jewish professionals and teach them trades — working with machines, simple carpentry, locksmithing.

Money was tight. Their first child, Frederick, was born. Edi had to work longer hours at harder jobs to support them. His cough worsened. And then, like a small boat dropping over a fall, Austria changed forever for Jews. The Night of Crystal, or Kristallnacht, was named for the sound of broken glass. A German soldier was killed by a rebel in France and the Nazis took to the streets in Germany and Austria claiming to seek retribution. They destroyed shopfronts, temples, and eateries. Nana and Edi hid in their apartment watching the terror from the window. It was clear that organized violence against Jews was escalating. The Gestapo were rounding some people up.

The rumors grew. There were places called labor camps where they were taking Jews. Julius, my great-uncle, was seized and taken to Dachau and later Buchenwald. Edi applied for jobs in England, but the laws covering immigration posed a challenge. Adults could emigrate, but children had to have English sponsors who would vouch for their well-being. Nana and Edi didn't know anyone in England, but they were desperate. They decided to separate. He would go ahead to England and send for her when he found a sponsor. He was put in touch with an English engineer and said he would work for almost nothing. He was hired.

The work was hard. He and many other young men from Vienna set to work clearing and renovating a barracks. There weren't many English people around, but Edi befriended a man who trucked food into the compound. He was willing to be a sponsor. Nana and Fred left for England as soon as they had the papers.

By 1940 the war was raging. They settled in Coventry, an industrial town of about 250,000 people on the Sherborne River a few hours by train from London. Narrow streets, old houses, crumbling town walls, and remains of old churches were vestiges of its fourteenth-century origin. For most of 1940, London was the primary target of German bombers, so Coventry seemed safe. There were many factories in the town and Edi was able to find work easily. Within a week his talents were recognized and he was made a line supervisor. It felt good to be there. His skills with machinery were in demand; he would help destroy the Gestapo with his brain and spirit. More than anything it was nice that no one asked if they were Jews. They were safe. Nana became pregnant and they welcomed Ann, my mother, into the world.

As the bombings in London intensified, some of the English became wary of recent German immigrants. The English were unaware that Jews from Austria and Germany were not loyal Germans. In July, a few months after my mother's birth, a sergeant appeared at Edward and Nana's apartment. He apologized for what he was there to do. He told Edward he would have to come with him. German and Austrian men were being taken to relocation camps. Some would be sent to Australia. Others would be taken north. Edward went peacefully. It would only be a setback, he told Nana.

I looked up the things Nana told me. Winston Churchill described the air raids on Coventry in detail in his book *The Second World War: Their Finest Hour.* In November of 1940 German strategists changed tactics. They shifted targets from London to other cities. They picked industrial centers. Special squads of airmen were trained to use new navigation machines. Cities like Glasgow, with its Rolls-Royce aero-engine works, and Coventry, with its munitions and aircraft factories, were targeted. On November 14, 1940, five hundred bombers attacked Coventry. Six hundred tons of high explosives and thousands of incendiaries were dropped. Four hundred people were killed. When the raid started, Ilse gathered her children and hid with them under the stairs in the makeshift shelter Edi had built. One of the children was crying. It was cold. There was a blanket upstairs, it would only take a moment. She was at the top of the stairs when the bomb landed. German radios later pronounced that Britian's other cities would be similarly "Coventrated."

In the internment camp in Scotland, Edi got word that Nana had suffered a head injury and was hospitalized. His children had been found two days after the bombings when Civil Defense Service workers went door to door in the bombed apartments looking for victims and survivors. Like many, the apartment was badly damaged. It was roofless and had no utilities. Edi was released and rushed back to his family. Ilse would be okay. He quickly set up tins to catch rainwater. Nana made new clothing for the children, using scraps of fabric from the old curtains. They would make do.

In the winter inclement weather kept them safe from the bombers. They repaired the apartment roof, heat was restored, and life returned to a semblance of normalcy. The radio reported that the enemy was targeting harbors. Cardiff, Portsmouth, and Swansea were bombed. Edi returned to the factory when it was operational. Nana tended the children. The respite was brief.

In April of 1941 the bombings started again. The combination of long days in the factory and air raids at night left Edi weak and exhausted. His cough was terrible. He and Nana decided to flee, taking only the children, the baby carriage, and what could be carried. They went to Windermere and then Langdale, in the Lake District in Northern England, far away from the industrial complex.

There, an elderly Quaker couple learned of their plight and offered to help. With no children of their own they showered Nana and Edi with gifts. They helped them find a place to stay and arranged for a doctor to see Edi. The man listened to Edi's chest, pronounced him cured, telling him he needn't return. They found clothing for the children and slowed Edi down. "No need to work so hard, my boy, you're safe here."

When Nana and Edi were settled the elderly Quaker woman helped Ilse with her English. They wrote the doctor a letter. Edi coughed all the time, how could he be cured? The doctor's response, lengthy and absolute, came three weeks later. Edi had a terminal condition. A lung disorder. He would die of it. It was only a matter of time. She needn't tell Edi the truth.

When the war ended they stayed in England. There was no family left in Austria. All who could had fled. The rest had perished in camps like Auschwitz, Treblinka and Buchenwald. In Langdale they lived in a cottage on a river which generated their electricity. Before Edi arrived the electricity was erratic and the water was undrinkable. There were problems with the generator. Edi volunteered to fix it and the power became more consistent. He also built a filter for the water. The townsfolk gave him the job of caring for the generator and he worked other odd jobs as well, fixing equipment for local farmers in exchange for eggs and other war-rare commodities.

They were accepted, even welcomed. For three years after the war they were part of the community. In December of 1948 Ilse and Edi threw a Christmas party. Despite being Jewish, they wanted to celebrate the holiday observed by the people who'd saved them. Eighty people arrived, and they all packed into the small cottage.

A blizzard swept in fast. Nana remembers Edi saying they should close the windows so that my mother wouldn't blow away. The lights flickered and went out. Edi gathered a coat around him, coughed a few times, and headed out into the storm to fix the generator.

He was dead three weeks later.

Nana gave me enough money to fly to London. I worked there for six weeks in a hotel and a pub, earning enough to travel to the Lake District. When I was ready I took a train to Windermere and then hitched rides to Langdale, where Nana said Edi was buried. I was walking, backpacked and lost, in the small town when an elderly man wearing a flannel shirt and a fisherman's cap stopped me. "Are you lost?" he asked me. I explained why I was there and held up the pencil drawing of the cottage. He smiled and shook his head. Looked at me curiously. "It's been years since I've thought of Edward," he said.

"I was a boy when your grandfather lived here. Here . . ." He offered his hand to me and led me along a dirt road. We walked hand in hand up the road. Eventually he stopped and pointed. The cottage. It'd been added to and was now a condo. As we stood in front of it he described Edi to me. "He had a laugh, that one," he said. "Right, he could fix anything. I remember McAlister walked six miles when his tractor stopped to get your grandfather. He was a hard one, too, had seen some down times I remember, but he was a good man. He could make a joke, too." Then he pointed to a winding road. "You'll be wanting to see where he is now, you'll find him a mile down." He used a stick and etched a map in the dirt for me.

I thanked him and set off down the newly paved road, lined by old limestone walls. I had a strange feeling as I walked the road. It was the first place in the U.K. I'd been that looked like New England, my home. The winding roads felt familiar, as if I might happen into my own neighborhood with time. The limestone walls, the dense green willows and heavy air.

I turned at the tree, as instructed, and followed a muddy path up the hill. At the top there was a knoll of shrubs and another limestone wall. When I found a break in the wall, I stepped into a small cemetery. Old thin stones were bent this way and that, like theatergoers straining to get a better look. The graves formed small hills in front of the stones. The effect made the dead more present. I needed to watch my step, lest I trip over someone's mound.

It took me a while but I found it. Edi's stone had been well cared for, though it was tilted and the words had faded a little. *Edward Freiberger. Father of Ann and Frederick. Proud husband to*

Ilse. I sat down. A light rain started and I wondered what it was like that night as he headed out into the blizzard.

Did you cough when you walked? Had you noticed that you walked slower and found it harder to draw breath? Or did you feel invincible? Did you know you were dying? And thank you for saving my mother. For working so hard and never giving up hope.

And as I sat there with a hand on the stone, I wondered if I was resilient enough to survive a crucible myself. To find strength, like him, over and over, setback after setback, and not rest until I'd given it everything I had. I didn't think so.

Integrative Medicine

After a few months of chemotherapy, I decided it would make sense to expand my treatment horizons. I didn't trust conventional medicine's monopoly on treatment. I read a macrobiotic cookbook first. It sounded great. I would eat only foods that were nutritious and lacked preservatives. Then I read the part about only eating food grown within twenty-five miles of one's home. The only food I knew growing near my home was the zucchini in the backyard. My mother found the book and flipped through it enthusiastically.

"You could have zucchini, tomatoes, pumpkin, and maybe we'll have more luck with the beans this year."

I've never enjoyed vegetables. Actually, I loathe them. I've speculated that early in my childhood I was attacked by a large broccoli and don't remember the details because it was so traumatic. My mother continued, hunched over the colorful *New Macrobiotic You* cookbook. "Hmmmm, maybe we could expand the garden. You might like squash, too." She eagerly scanned the recipes.

Later I sat with my brother on the couch. His face was six inches from the pages of a J. R. R. Tolkien paperback. He said softly, still looking at the book, "So, which do you think will be worse, the chemotherapy or trying to subsist on Mom's garden?"

"I'll let you know," I told him.

"I'll sneak you hamburgers if you want," David offered.

I adhered for two weeks. The ill-fated diet came to a violent end one night when an unnamed figure bathed in refrigerator light desperately violated a pint of Ben & Jerry's with an oversized soup spoon.

Imagery was next. I ran into one of Mom's friends in Park Avenue Pizza. A short woman with scarred cheeks, she leaned toward me and whispered as if we were suburban spies, "Did you know Bobby Arnold's mother? She cured herself of cervical cancer with imagery. You must do it." I picked up a book on imagery and started practicing.

I imagined good cells attacking bad cells before I went to sleep every night. The cells started on opposite sides, lined up neatly, and then marched toward one another as if they were medieval knights. Once they got close together, I had a harder time controlling what happened. Sometimes the good cells and the bad cells behaved and stayed neat and organized, but other times they merged into a chaotic, writhing square dance gone terribly awry. Sometimes I tried to organize them, but most of the time I just went to sleep.

One of my father's colleagues sent him a book on tape. I listened to it in the car during my drive back to Vassar after a chemotherapy hit. The author was a surgeon at a prestigious hospital

who asserted that if cancer patients would simply think optimistically, they could destroy their cancers. It was a beautiful idea but
made me nervous. Had I been thinking the wrong way before? Is
that why I developed cancer? How come so many of the people I
knew who'd lived a long time were crotchety and often pessimistic, resembling Henry Fonda from *On Golden Pond*? I tried
to think optimistically.

Another book promised that imbibing shark cartilage would
keep away my illness. The logic asserted that swallowing a sub-
stance that does not get cancer would be magically protective. It
took "You are what you eat," a seventies mantra, to an exciting
new extreme. Then I thought about other things that don't get
cancer. Scissors. Cashmere. Asbestos. Not appetizing.

On a trip with friends into New York City, I found a homeo-
pathic Chinese medicine pharmacy. It was poorly lit and dusty. I
arrived at the counter after fighting through paper umbrellas and
ninja outfits. A little man sat at the counter reading a Chinese
paper. Behind him were hundreds of jars of varying shapes, colors,
and sizes labeled in Chinese on yellowing paper. I could see roots
and berries and pastes. They cluttered the shelves all the way to
the ceiling. A coworker whistled as he swept nearby. The man
behind the counter looked up at me. He had a wrinkled face and
one of his eyes was darker than the other. He was balding and had
a pleasant birthmark high on his forehead. I asked him if he had
anything for cancer. The coworker stopped sweeping. They both
stared at me. I wasn't sure if they understood me so I repeated
myself and spoke slower. "Ah!" the counterman muttered. He
turned and scanned the jars as if deep in thought. "Hmmmm," he
said. He scratched his birthmark. Then he slowly turned around,
looked at me gently, moved toward me, and took one of my hands
in his, patting it slowly. His eyes looked, unblinking, into mine. He
whispered, nodding his head, "See a doctor."

Cowboy Hats, Earrings, and Doctors

Scenes with my Father

Two Years Old

My mother is telling me to be quiet. My father has worked the night shift on the railroad. Even though it's morning, he's just gone to sleep. I don't know who he is exactly. He's left a gift for me. A cowboy hat. It hangs on an orange kitchen chair where my booster seat is tied. I like it. I am afraid he will wake up if I take it. My mother wants me to hold it but I won't. If I stand in one place and don't make a sound, maybe he won't wake up.

Five Years Old

My father is on his knees facing me. He's furious. I can see the tips of his two front teeth behind a quivering upper lip. He is scream-ing at me for tying up my little brother's hands with fishing line. "What were you thinking?" *I don't know. It was stupid. I could have hurt him.* I don't speak. "Look at me." I wonder, Did I really want to hurt him? *Maybe I did. I'm bad.*

The emotion wells up and out of me and I'm shaking and gasping for air. He holds me. Tight. "Danny, you have to think before you do things. He's smaller than you. It's okay. You didn't realize what you were doing." He is saying, "Your brother is fine. Just don't do that again. It's okay." *It's okay.*

Six Years Old

It's been a long car ride, three hours from Hartford to Newark. My brother and I fell asleep long ago, but now I'm in the soft gap between asleep and awake. I recognize the sounds of our street. The car is slowing and the street lamps send long yellow lines across the fabric on the ceiling of the car and the back of my mother's seat. We are turning into our driveway. I don't need to look, I know this. I recognize the bump where the street and driveway meet. I hear my mother gathering things from around her feet. The engine stalls silent. For a moment there's nothing. Then my mother says something. My father forgot to put away the push mower before we left. It could rust.

I could get up now. I'm big enough to climb down out of the seat, open my door, and walk across the yard and up the back staircase into the house. But I don't. I keep my eyes closed. With the motor off the world is near quiet. Even here in Newark, in the city, there are crickets in our little backyard. The car door opens next to me. A hand burrows beneath me. I am lifted and wrapped into my father, my face pressed against his thin T-shirt. I can smell him, oil and soap, sweat and life. I am lifted out of the car. I hear his footsteps up the back stairs beneath me, the screen door opening and the familiar groan of the back door, swollen from the summer humidity. I don't want him to put me in my bed. I want to stay right here, sleep the rest of the night buried in his chest.

Eight Years Old

It was going to be a perfect sledding run. We'd only just moved to Connecticut and I was enjoying my first heavy snowfall. I'd hit top speed and then glide under the soccer posts. Lee, my friend, had a running start and leapt onto his sled. He went fast, hitting a small jump and then flying through the posts and gliding another thirty feet before stopping. I tucked my jacket into my gloves. Ran my gloves down my jeans and brushed off the snow. My legs were getting cold. Lee stood at the bottom of the hill and taunted me. He bet I couldn't get as far. He'd see.

I aligned my sled and paced off fifteen steps uphill. I ran as fast as I could while still maintaining control and jumped, chest down onto the sled. I landed cleanly and the sled jerked into motion. I hit the bump perfectly, accelerating, lifting and landing evenly. Then the patch of ice. The right runner caught something and I was careening toward one of the posts. It came on fast. *Roll off?* I held my hands out in front of me.

Shearing pain. I looked up and my finger was in the wrong place, up high on my hand. I screeched. Yanked off the glove. Someone's father hustled me up the hill and toward my house. The man rang our bell and my father answered. Saw my hand. The man seemed panicked. My father surveyed the hand, thanked the man, and told my brother to get some ice. Then he walked me out to the car. He slowly opened the door and told me to get in. He was humming something. My brother came out with ice in a towel and he handed it to me. I sat in the back with ice pressed against my hand. Dad wrote a note to my mom and slipped it into the front door, made my brother get our jackets, belted him in front, and drove us to the hospital.

He looked at me in the rearview mirror every now and then. Smiling. "You okay, Champ?" Calm.

Ten Years Old

We are forty miles outside of Jefferson City. I know this because I have been following the maps. Today Dad drove eleven hundred miles, farther than we'd planned by three hundred miles. He's exhausted, but going fast saved us some time and by tomorrow afternoon we'll be camping in the Rockies. The motel was full. Dad talked the manager into allowing us to use a room that's usually used by a housekeeper. It has only one bed.

Me, David, and Mom snuggle into the bed. Dad makes a bed out of a few sweaters and a chair cushion on the floor. Mom tells him he deserves the bed. He's driven all day. What about his back? He tells her to sleep in the bed. He'll be fine. His voice leaves no room for negotiation. I don't want to sleep on the floor, but I don't say anything. They turn out the light.

Twelve Years Old

We are outside shoveling. More snow has accumulated in northern Connecticut than at any time in the last fifty-four years. The air is thick with heavy flakes and my wrists, where my gloves meet my coat, are wet. The snow is up to my head, my father's shoulders. I am almost as tall as I will get, but my father still stands a head taller. His shoulders are broad and he swings his shovel consistently, a breath in, a breath out, swing and throw, swing and throw. My methods are more inconsistent. I push some. I throw some. I carry and heave. Down near the street where the driveway ends, there is a tall crusty pile from the snowplow. For a while we work back to back. David is doing the front stairs. He is meticulous, working each stair one at a time. But down here we do the heavy work. When we're finished my father pulls off his hat and scarf and stands surveying our work. Taps me on the shoulder. "Nice work, Champ." Pride rises in my chest. I pull off my hat and brush the water from my cheeks. I want to catch a snowflake in my mouth, but I'll wait until he goes inside.

Thirteen Years Old

Dad has driven me to our local pharmacy. He hasn't told me why. He walks with purpose toward the back counter. I follow him.

"Hi, Bob," my father greets the pharmacist.

"Hi, Mr. Shapiro, what can we do for you today?"

"Bob, I want you to show my son here the condoms," my father says. I can feel my eyebrows lifting.

"Certainly, Mr. Shapiro," says Bob, as if this is common. Bob turns behind him, pulls one of each type of condom from the shelf and drops it on the counter in front of me. There are black and red and blue boxes. Bob clears his throat, pushes his glasses higher on his nose and begins, as if they are insects and he the head entomologist. He describes each one's genus and mechanism like when we went to the children's science museum in Boston.

Bob points. "These are sheep skinned and lubricated, and these, over here, are latex—that's a type of rubber, hence the vernacular—also ribbed. Over here, these are the least expensive but also have a reservoir tip, unribbed, not lubricated. Incidentally, reservoir tips can be very important." And on and on. At first I try to pretend he's talking about something else. But I look up at my father, who's biting his lip, and just at that moment Bob says the word *lubricated* and it sounds funny. I giggle. My father's shoulders lift and fall and I think he's laughing, too, but I don't look at him. Bob pretends I haven't laughed. He continues, without missing a beat, and I manage to make it through the rest of the short presentation without collapsing or having a seizure. At the end Dad looks at me and says, "Any questions?" and I shake my head, no, and he says, "I truly appreciate this, Bob," and we walk out. On the way home I stare out my window and don't speak.

Nineteen Years Old

I've just been voted president of my dorm at Vassar as a write-in candidate. Dad is picking me up. I've pierced my ear since he saw me last and I'm looking forward to shocking him. I borrowed a bright red Christmas ball from the dorm tree and I'm wearing it in my ear. His Chevy pulls in behind my dorm. I throw my bags in the trunk and get into the car. I swing my head so the earring bounces from my cheek to my neck and back. He looks at me. Flat. "How were your exams?" he asks. No other response. Damn. I pull the earring from my ear and the corners of his mouth turn upward. Then he smirks, shakes his head no, and by the time we drive out of Vassar's main gate, we are laughing and laughing.

Twenty-One Years Old

When chemotherapy was over and it was time to start radiation treatments, I was prepared. I realized already that some physicians share everything they know, all speculations and even guesses, while others offer only the crumbs they're certain about. I thought it was a mistake to assume that physicians would tell me what I needed to know. I'd probably have to ask questions. The hard questions in particular.

I asked for a meeting with the radiation oncologist before I started the fifteen treatments. In total I'd be getting twenty-four hundred rads of radiation, roughly five hundred times the amount in an X ray. In high school I watched a documentary about children who'd been just outside ground zero when the atomic bomb landed in Nagasaki. Radiation made me nervous. My father came along and sat between us, quietly, in the little room with bright fluorescent lights and the glossy poster of flowers on the wall.

I was shrewd and prepared. I fired question after question at the

little doctor, trying to disarm him by letting him know I was knowl-
edgeable. I would not be evaded. I wanted to force him to tell me
every side effect, every nuance of treatment. I asked every question I
could think of, "I know radiation can cause pulmonary difficulties,
what will you do to prevent those?" and "Will I have permanent
cardiac problems?" and "What's gonna happen to my spine?"

He seemed forthcoming. When he wasn't sure he said so and
I felt I could trust him. I relaxed and asked about more immediate
side effects—nausea, sore throat, fatigue and weight loss. I was
midsentence when I heard a guttural sob and looked.

My father was doubled over, trembling. His shoulders shook
and his hands covered his face. I saw a dark spot, a drop of water
on his loafers. I looked back at the doc, set my jaw, and continued
my questioning—I didn't reach for my father, I didn't touch him.
While my dad sobbed and shook I asked about hair loss and skin
burns, scheduling and parking. The doctor quietly answered each
question. And we, the doctor and me, played out our charade as if
nothing was happening, both of us ill-equipped to do anything
but be doctor and patient.

Lime

The machine started. It hummed, loud, and every hair on my
body stood up, but then they relaxed and I realized it was just
nerves. The technician had aligned me carefully on the table,
matching tattoos on my chest with red laser beams generated
from across the room. It felt very futuristic, the darkened room
and red lasers, the hushed technicians and hovering machines.
When she had me just right she told me not to move and left the
room. I waited. Then the machine started and a buzzer sounded.

It was loud and unrelenting. It reminded me of the buzzers in World War II movies that signaled a submarine was diving. The sound suggested that something important was happening.

A minute later it stopped. She reappeared. "That's it," she said. Two hundred and seventy rads down, only twenty-one hundred to go. I climbed off the table, put my T-shirt back on, and headed out to the parking lot. It was autumn; I was finally finished with chemotherapy and life was starting to look up. I'd heard I might burn a little from the radiation, like a sunburn, or have a parched throat, but compared to the side effects of chemotherapy, this would be a breeze. When we spoke about the radiation, my parents had been concerned. None of us had any experience with radiation or its side effects outside of PBS documentaries about Madame Curie, or Hiroshima and Nagasaki, or that atoll in the South Pacific that we kept bombing.

On the drive back to my parents' house, I stopped at a hardware store. I searched for a while, comparing spray paint colors and talking to a kid I knew from high school who worked there. I told him what I was looking for and why and he laughed. Then he disappeared into the back room. When he reappeared, with the same jaunt he had used when coming in late to Chemistry, he was shaking the can in one hand and had an empty cardboard box in the other.

"We can't sell this color to save our lives," he started. "Check this out." And he aimed the can at a cardboard box and sprayed. It left a wide circle on the box. It was perfect. The color of the pulp inside a lime but brighter. "It's Neon Lime," he said, beaming. "I could probably hook you up with some Evergreen, too, but I don't think it's as bright and it ain't on sale." I took the Neon Lime.

In the car again I rolled the can along the passenger seat. I imagined my mother's response. I'd approach her, my hands clutching my chest, and plead, "Ma, what's happening to me?"

"OHMYGOD," she might gasp. "HOW TERRIBLE!" Her

mouth hanging open. She might rush to the phone and call the head of radiation oncology.

At home I greeted my mother, "Hey, Ma," and headed downstairs.

"How'd it go?" came her voice from upstairs, but I didn't respond. My bedroom was just outside the garage on the first floor. The kitchen and other bedrooms were upstairs. I stepped inside the garage, cleared a spot next to the lawn mower, and sat down. Took off my shirt. I shook the can and then sprayed some on my chest, starting in the middle and making light concentric circles outward until the "radiation field," roughly the upper half of my torso, was lime green. It was cold in the garage and the fumes were strong. I took a newspaper from the trash pile and fanned it over my chest, waiting for it to dry. It took a while. Then I put on an old oxford shirt and climbed the stairs.

I found Mom in the living room. She was hanging a large framed sketch of a clown, drawn completely with one line, on the wall. More odd folk art.

I said it as I'd practiced it. Urgent. My voice even quivered a little.

"Ma! What's happening to me?!" I pleaded, throwing open my shirt and dramatically revealing my lime green chest. I turned my head up toward the ceiling for effect.

She looked down at my chest. Then up.

"Lime suits your eyes." She looked back at the clown. "Is this straight?" she asked. As she adjusted it she added, "You know, you might have them radiate the rest of you. It really is a fine shade of green." She paused, then said, "I hope you didn't get paint on anything in your bedroom."

"I was careful," I answered. "Hey, if I try this on David and Dad, you won't say anything, will you?"

"No, dear, you go right ahead and terrify the family."

"Thanks, Ma," and I headed off for my brother's bedroom.

Dice

Seventy percent survival over five years. That's pretty good, right? I mean, those are great odds. Especially since it was 100 percent fatal just twenty years ago. But what if I'm in the 30 percent group? Can't think that. Can't even let that thought in. I have to be in the 70 percent. Don't I? And it's 70 percent for my staging, right, not just for this particular disease. But I've got heavy disease—I mean, even the docs were saying they hadn't seen a tumor that large in someone's chest. So I've got more of a chance of being in the 30 percent . . . don't even think that. Where's the Yahtzee game? It's got dice in it. Okay, 70 percent multiplied by 12 is 8.4, so 8 and above means I'm in the 30 percent group, and 7 and below means I'm in the 70 percent group. Deep breath. Roll. Ugh. A 9. Maybe it's best out of three. That's better. A 6. And again to decide everything. A 10. Oh no. Maybe it's best out of five?

Wait a minute. There's no such thing as a 70 percent chance of surviving for five years for one individual. There's either a 100 percent chance or a 0 percent chance. I won't be 70 percent alive. I'll be either alive or dead. Period. No matter what.

People keep telling me about other people they've known with Hodgkin's disease. Dad called me to the television when the Saturday-afternoon movie showed Robert De Niro portraying a guy dying of Hodgkin's who played catcher for the Yankees. David showed me the sports page; Paul Allen, the owner of the Portland Trailblazers, had it. A friend's oldest brother had it, and Wans, the guy who told me about marijuana, and people's aunts and cousins and bosses and on and on. All of a sudden a disease I'd never heard of was everywhere.

We can't all be in the 70 percent group, can we?

Literary Therapy

Before my diagnosis I'd accumulated a pile of paperbacks I wanted to read over the summer. They were by psychologists, psychiatrists, and science fiction writers. There was Stephen King and Erving Goffman, J. R. R. Tolkien and Irvin Yalom.

Then, after I was diagnosed, a friend gave me a self-help book with a title resembling *Think Your Way to Health*. It reminded me of those "do-it-yourself" books, how to build your own deck, hot tub, or doghouse. Like those books, which inevitably showed a workman cutting a perfect circle in a wall with a handsaw, this one also had a message that was too simple.

Still, I looked at my ambitious pile of nonfiction and escapist paperbacks and realized I wasn't interested in them anymore. I started looking for firsthand accounts of struggle. I didn't care how literary they were, as long as the writing was clear and I could get a glimpse of how people coped with challenge. I read *All Quiet on the Western Front, Papillon,* and the *Letters of Sacco and Vanzetti* — anything I could find that portrayed anguish and a response to it. My professors and friends helped. Anne Constantinople, a passionate social psychology professor, searched her tall oak bookcase, a finger drumming on her lip, and pulled out a Dostoyevsky collection. Ken Levine, a close friend, handed over a biography of Gandhi. "Gandhi's the man," he said. And my new pile grew. Jack London. Fitzgerald. Vonnegut.

I read while waiting to get chemotherapy and during lunch and late at night. Papillon lived in solitary confinement for five years, surviving by focusing on staying healthy and avoiding self-pity. Sacco and Vanzetti were sentenced to death and then executed for crimes they didn't commit. They thrived by writing, which led them to find a greater purpose in their deaths. And the children in Hiroshima, the Warsaw ghetto fighters, the long marchers across China, and those trapped by winter ice in Antarctica. Even the British, French, and German kids, living across from one another in trenches during the First World War, locked in what felt like a meaningless battle.

Though the books never revealed where the strength came from, in each story there was a handful of people who clawed a path toward thriving, even in the midst of overwhelming horrors. They clenched their fists, found a greater purpose, disciplined themselves, and followed a realistic, determined hopefulness.

Dad's Clarinet

There are sounds from my childhood I'll never forget. Heavy footsteps above. The sound of the closet door opening in my father's study, the heavy drag of the door pulled over shag carpet, and then the scrape of a wooden case lifted from a shelf. Then I'd hear him in the kitchen, pacing while he held the reed in his mouth, wetting the wood. I'd hear the radio go off, National Public Radio's constant sound—*Bob and Ray*, or *Prairie Home Companion*, or *All Things Considered*—replaced with an uncommon silence. And then, eventually, the first sounds. A few simple notes. A scale or two. Then pacing again, a little faster, impatient, because the reed wasn't ready.

In his yearbook I found out that Dad was called "the Benny Goodman of Weaver High" by his classmates. He was "All New England" and used to give performances in places like Boston and Philadelphia. He could sight-read anything—jazz, classical, blues.

When we were growing up Dad didn't pull out the clarinet very often. Still doesn't. I'm not sure why. My father had such a level spirit, like a wide rowboat in flat water, only the occasional ripple escaped. But there were rare times of passion, rage or laughter. And happiness, marked most clearly when he had the instrument in his hands. The world had to be right for him to pull it out. Most notably, Mom had to be in a good mood. Bills paid. Chores completed. My brother and I on good terms with the universe. Once every few months he'd stride into his study and reappear with the little black case.

Inside, after you flip up the perfectly aligned clasps, there's purple velvet holding each of the ebony parts. Each reed lives inside its own slot as if it were a kitchen knife in butcher block. Each black, mystical part has its own darker, worn-velvet home like the dip in a well-used mattress. Dad keeps the reed in his mouth while he twists together the parts, pressing down silver levers with long fingers. And then the first notes. "Still not ready," he says, standing and walking with the instrument.

After a little while longer he'd really start. Jazz and blues, his clarinet dropping riffs like bright autumn leaves. Optimistic yellows and mourning reds and haunting oranges. As he blew the clarinet, his eyebrows lifted, and he nodded and shook his head with each riff as if he were in a passionate conversation.

I loved to watch him with it. He'd sometimes look at me while he played, as if each note were a piece of advice, or a shared confidence. He could joke with it, use a scale to ask a question, or tease with seven notes running up like a predictable staircase only to drop through a trapdoor at the top. He could scowl and prance and laugh. I guess more than anything, though, he could celebrate. Use jazz riffs as a steam whistle, a stint releasing our pressures.

———

I believed that my last radiation treatment was the end of my cancer experience. I drove home afterward and buried myself in my room. Treatment was finally over. No more chemotherapy. No more radiation. I thought I'd feel an unburdening, that feeling of getting home on a cold icy night, but I didn't. There was a nervousness. From now on I'd have to live not knowing if the disease was going to come back.

I tossed and turned in my bed, unable to relax. Eventually I just stared at the ceiling, my hands crossed on my chest. In my college-aged self-centeredness it didn't occur to me that my last treatment was significant for the entire family. I heard their voices upstairs, carrying like pieces of paper on a breeze.

Then I heard my father's footsteps on the linoleum floor above, the first few notes and his muffled voice, "Still not ready." I sat up and listened. Nothing. And then the familiar sound, a few easy riffs, and then it broke open. My father's voice singing through the clarinet, whooping and hollering in celebration. And sudden images of chemotherapy—the needles and smell of alcohol, steel I.V. poles and plastic-covered recliners—all of it flooded back and released to his serenade. No more. No more.

Dictated Chart Note

11/87

The patient underwent six cycles of MOPP chemotherapy followed by 2400cGy of mantle radiation. Sequential X-rays throughout the course of therapy noted a marked reduction in the size of the mediastinal mass and complete resolution of his lymphadenopathy. In addition the patient showed a complete resolution of B symptoms following two cycles of MOPP chemotherapy. At completion of therapy a chest CT revealed some residual mass, however it is our opinion that this represents scar only and the patient is in a complete remission. Given his stage and responsiveness to therapy, this patient has a 70% chance for long term, disease free, survival.

CHARLES BRODSKY, M.D.
St. Francis Medical Center

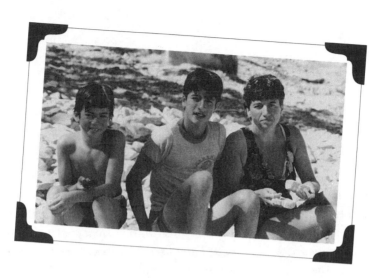

Part Two

Transitions

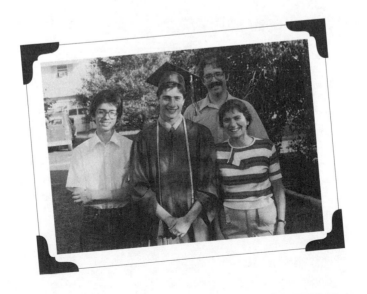

Dictated Chart Note

6/90

This is a healthy appearing 22-year-old Caucasian male with a history of Stage IIB nodular sclerosing Hodgkin's disease who presented with a four week history of persistent cervical lymphadenopathy. A 4 cm. matted and fixed left cervical node was palpated. The patient has been referred to the surgical team for nodal biopsy.

CHARLES ERIC SCHULMAN, M.D.
Shands Hospital at the University of Florida

Red Line Magic

I graduated from Vassar and was accepted in a clinical psychology Ph.D. program at the University of Florida. Cancer and chemotherapy quickly faded from memory, eclipsed by graduate school applications, final exams, and good-byes.

That summer I lived in Boston with Eric, Jay, and Chuck, friends from Vassar. One particular Saturday morning, Eric and I wandered down the Red Line stairs, through the turnstiles, and deep into the long corridor to wait for the train. We'd only settled onto a bench for a moment when we heard faint music. Chimes. They started softly and grew louder and louder, gathering around us, a rich, melodic vibrato singing through the tunnel, echoing down the tiles and along the shiny tracks. Perhaps it was because of the humid tiles, or maybe the tunnel had unique acoustics, but to me it was a sound that could have competed with the bells of Notre Dame.

We searched for the source. Speakers? A sophisticated boom box? Eventually we noticed an old woman standing across the tracks, on the Boston-bound side of the Red Line. She wore a kerchief on her head and had a shopping bag at her thick knees. Gray shoots of hair framed a windblown, seasoned face. She was cranking a small handle that stuck out of the wall. My eyes followed the thin steel rods up the wall and across the dark, sooty concrete ceiling, to long steel tubes that hung between the tracks. I hadn't even noticed them. I looked down our side and saw a

49

young black man cranking a similar handle. He wore athletic shorts and a muscle shirt; his arms looked strong and capable. He held a paperback in his other large hand.

Together the strangers' efforts rang the chimes. When I looked back at the old woman, I noticed she was laughing at the resonating sound and cranking harder. They played and played and played until our train roared into the station and stopped with a squeal. The doors slid open and we got on. Through the window I watched the old woman gather her bag, and a walking stick I'd missed, and hobble slowly toward a bench. The black man boarded and sat near us, burying his face in his book.

That experience stayed with me, became a talisman, like a gemstone carried on a key ring or a poem kept in a wallet. It got stored with other pleasant memories that revisit me at odd times, water streaming like beads of mercury across a windowpane during an autumn thunderstorm, the thwacking sound of flip-flops a few sizes too big, or the smell of fresh-baked bagels.

Bringing myself to the hospital later would be an act of faith. I entrusted my body, my life's only vehicle, to strangers. Strangers whose attitudes and ethics I could not assess. Lying on gurneys, in waiting rooms, in hospital beds, and under scanners, I'd often worry. *What if they don't care enough and just screw this up? What if they're having a bad day?* But then I'd settle on the memory of a summer morning in Boston and strangers' music echoing down the Red Line tracks.

Really Deep Intellectual Courtship

I'm walking into the bone marrow transplant unit. The nursing director, Ms. Terry Wikle, stops me. Who am I there to see? she wants to know. She's in her late twenties or early thirties. Beautiful. Long brown hair. Brown eyes. Slight features. She wears dangling earrings and soft lipstick, business dress instead of nursing wear. She moves with confidence, like a teenager in her childhood room. She asks if I'm a medical student. I sense she does not respect medical students. I tell her I'm from clinical psychology and am going to visit Jodi, my first patient. She lets me pass.

A few days later, I'm camping out in her office. How long could she be? The other graduate students and I have been warned by our chairman that we're taking too long to complete the Ph.D. program. The national average is five years. In our program it takes most students seven years. We must get started on our master's thesis research projects immediately or some of us will be weeded out. One has left already. I don't want to do a study of college students. I want to study something important. Maybe I will study how people cope when they're on the bone marrow transplant unit?

Nurse Wikle appears and eyes me skeptically. Sits down and picks up her appointment book. What am I doing in her office? I tell her I want to talk to her about research. She puts down the appointment book. Stares at me. Smiles.

"Well, aren't you business, business, business," she mocks. "I tell you what, Mr. Research, here's my home number. Call me. We'll go out for drinks and talk aaaaaaaalllllll about your research."

She hands me a piece of paper. *Hello?*

I call a few nights later and get her answering machine. When Terry returns the call, she says, "I'll tell you what we're doing, Mr. Research, and you decide if you want to come. Whenever one of my nurses leaves the unit we celebrate wherever they want. Anywhere, understand? So Phil is leaving and we're going to Club Paradise. Have you been to Club Paradise?"

A few hours later I see my very first pierced nipples. On a guy. Phil. He shows them to me soon after I arrive, lifting up his turtleneck to reveal two shining silver hoops. "Very nice," I tell him.

"You wanna get yours done?" he asks me.

Then a big man with a beard trots over and asks him to dance. Phil winks at me and is gone. Another man appears a moment later, short, with wire-rim glasses and a nice vest. He asks me to dance. "He's taken, sweetie," Terry says, appearing and draping an arm around me.

"Fag hag," the man mutters.

"Bitch," Terry responds. Then she smiles at me. "I didn't know you were such a tease." The bar is smoky and loud and the clientele is as varied as the music. There's leather and flashing lights, some men in suits and others in little shorts. "Come on," Terry says, and she leads me onto the crowded dance floor where I let the bass and synthesizers drive.

Later that night, we're in an all-night pizza place. I notice a video game, Galaga. I've played it since it first came out and I know all the tricks. Galaga is an art.

"Hey," I say casually. "There's a Galaga machine."

"Oh?" she asks. Uninterested.

"Wanna play while we wait for the food?" I ask.

"I guess."

And there we are standing in front of the machine. I put in two quarters so we both can play. I go first. I do reasonably well for me, getting easily through the first couple rounds before I'm assaulted by an alien space pod that curls on top of me. Terry asks how the controls work. I show her, standing behind her for the first few moments. Pressed against her. Her hair smells of smoke and lilacs. Then she takes over. The aliens start simply, coming at her from only two directions. She mows them down. Luck. I compliment her. The aliens line up for round two. Again she mows them down. Now the aliens are angry. They dodge and weave, assaulting her from all angles. But she is resilient and her wrist snaps with agility. Her forefinger presses the firing button quickly. Soon her score approaches mine. Then passes it. And on. Now the aliens give it everything they have, decoying with a slow alien while another zips in from the far side of the screen. No luck. Now another three drop in at once, leaving her nowhere to move, but she survives. Then they all drop in on her, firing and whizzing. Soon she has the high score.

I am in love.

Deep into the morning we are kissing and writhing on her living-room floor when she whispers, "Good things come to those who wait."

I boast, "I hope you can be patient," and we giggle and giggle and giggle.

I didn't know, wouldn't know for years, that Terry heard the first warning two days after our first date. Paula Lee, a cherub nurse who'd danced the night away with us, talked to Terry during

the shift change. She'd heard about my illness from a friend. "You
know about Hodgkin's disease," she said. "He could die, you know.
I know someone else, he's cute and healthy and the two of you
would get along so well. . . ." Terry thanked her for her concern.
And there were others, nurses and doctors, aides and secretaries,
who told her they cared about her. They didn't want to see her get
involved in something that couldn't go anywhere.

As I got to know her I studied her carefully. Terry swung her arms
when she walked, as if she owned the land around her. Her fear-
lessness was as steady as the chimes on my grandfather's desk
clock. She reminded me of the star runner on our high-school
track team, Granger, who used to look at the finish line with the
calm acceptance that it was his. Terry wore that same expression
no matter what she faced. I'd later see it as we leapt into a tossing
black ocean, getting certified to scuba dive. And as she merged
her aging Volvo into an intersection flooded from a downpour,
speeding tractor trailers roaring through a gray squall. And again
as she ran out of her office, holding her stethoscope to her chest, a
patient code buzzer sounding the alarm.

The patient emergencies were particularly revealing. Her
friends teased her about her calm during emergencies. How well
she ran codes. None of the nurses were as composed when a
patient's systems teetered. I imagined her doing the whole thing
herself, running for the crash cart, pushing in epinephrine,
checking airways.

Terry was six years older than me. She had been married.
Divorced. Her first husband was an airline pilot, more comfortable in the air than on the ground. When he piloted his life he
avoided all trying weather, all dark clouds, all lightning and wind.
When she brought up problems, routine relationship mainte-
nance, he reminded her that things were okay, no need to worry,
why make a fuss? We're cloudless, after all.

I met Terry a few months after their separation. I was just twenty-two, a graduate student. A glorified college student really. I had a one-bedroom apartment replete with a yellow couch that might have been featured in a 1965 Lord & Taylor catalog, which would have been fine, but it was 1988. I had a stringy, second-hand rug and a black-and-white television that preferred PBS to all other channels and would occasionally shut off and need a thirty-minute rest if something really engaging was on. I ate ramen noodles from the pot I cooked them in. Five meals for a dollar. Food. In the bedroom I built a platform out of plywood and dropped a futon on it. Bed. Added an unfinished door over two file cabinets. Desk.

Terry, in contrast, owned a small house near the hospital. I walked by it every day. When she cooked for me, she served stuffed chicken breasts with lemon asparagus on real china that had floral patterns. She had framed Matisse and Manet reproductions. A carpeted living room with a matching "L" sofa and love seat. She had a bed with a real backboard and a place to put books and a built-in reading light. There were bookcases filled with stories of quirky characters—Armistead Maupin's *Tales of the City*, Salinger's *Franny and Zooey*, and Tom Robbins's *Even Cowgirls Get the Blues*. Her home smelled of potpourri and a hint of perfume. Mine smelled of sneakers.

My favorite feature in her house was the porch. She had a screened-in porch with a hanging love seat that looked out over a groomed yard and the road. A little bird lived on the porch, her pet cockatiel. Whenever I walked by on my way into the hospital, the bird whistled to me, and I back, and he scurried along the base of the screen door, his little yellow tuft of hair bobbing up and down.

One night while we were out at a hospital function, I watched Terry from across the room, her long frizzy hair surrounding her, and I realized that she wore adulthood like a seductive fragrance. I knew then that I wanted to bury my head under her chin and hold on, and dance, and sway, and laugh, and love.

Blue Towels

The little house where Terry lived was too small. No place for me
to set up a desk. My apartment wasn't even considered. So we
looked together. We asked apartment managers about counter-
space, closets, and cats. A few weeks later I found myself, for the
first time as a young adult, in a new furniture store. I'd always
found my dorm or grad school furniture in used establishments.
And not just any. I went to the cheapest. Dusty, cluttered places
that were as much graveyard as display.

Now I stood in a store with high ceilings and carpeting. The
salespeople had name tags and clipboards, fabric swatches and
colored fold-out dining set descriptions. We were looking at a
massive leather pit-group. I took off my loafers and hopped on. It
was far more supportive than my Lord and Taylor model and it
was huge. I smiled. It was great! Terry pinched a pillow and asked
about stains and warranties. A few minutes later we surveyed coffee tables. Big glass beasts with brass legs and "compelling lines,"
as the saleswoman explained. Terry looked at me and asked my
opinion. "You know, coffee tables are my specialty," I offered.
Terry raised an eyebrow, pointed at one and said she'd write a
check. In twenty minutes we spent the equivalent of three months
of my graduate student salary. When I saw the total, I looked at
Terry. "Don't worry, kiddo," she said, "I'm buying. Next time we
buy a couch, dining room table, and coffee table, it's on you."

A few days later we sat in the Lakewood Villas management
office and paid the first and last month for a lease for a two-
bedroom loft. It was new. It had a porch and new kitchen and I'd
have my own office. After they gave us the keys we walked in

together. It felt like a joke. I wasn't an adult. I couldn't possibly live here yet.

The morning we unpacked we worked on different parts of the apartment. I set up my office, trying to keep all of my graduate materials organized. When I took a break I walked into my new bathroom and found that Terry had already been there. There were matching blue towels and washcloths, potpourri, candles, and even a little blue soap. I looked down and found I was standing on a matching blue bath rug.

After I dried my hands I straightened the towel and took a few extra moments to line it up with the other one and the washcloth. Swallowed. This was going to be very different.

Mom's Marijuana: Part C

The Gainesville airport is small. It doesn't even have a tower. There are two gates and you can see both from the airport lobby. It's a humid night, the air heavy with sweat and the occasional mosquito. Gainesville is a college town and the airport is filled with college wear. There are a lot of baseball caps, ponytails, and shorts. People sit reading or watching tiny televisions built into kiosks scattered through the lobby.

Football is on television. I'm watching the second half of a depressing Patriots game when I see their plane coast down outside the windows. I stand up with the others and we gather around the gate. Then, a little while later, I feel a familiar comfort as I spot my father's bobbing bald head. And then Mom. That confident stride I'd know anywhere. Her purse strap runs across her body like a crossing guard's reflector and for a moment she looks as if she's in uniform. Before I realize it I'm cutting through the small crowd and into their arms. Both of them at once. Big tired smiles. My cheeks feel hot.

We stand quietly at the baggage conveyor. A few bags arrive and we pull them off the belt. Then more. And more. Mom has never been an efficient packer. It's more important to be prepared for any eventuality than to be able to fit one's luggage into a standard-sized vehicle like, say, a U-Haul. The sixth bag arrives. It's roughly the size of a Buick.

"Jimmy Hoffa's body is in there?" my father suggests.

"Don't be a wise-ass," my mother says. I grunt under the weight.

The inquisition starts on the drive. My parents haven't been to Gainesville before. Or our new apartment. Is there any place to get good bagels in this town? Is the biopsy still scheduled for Thursday morning? How long will I be in the hospital? Since I haven't had any other symptoms, couldn't it just be a cyst or something? I look tired — have I been going to classes? Do I want my father to drive? Maybe I shouldn't have carried the bags? How's graduate school, is it harder than Vassar?

Dad and I lug the baggage into our new apartment. We carry in the Jimmy Hoffa bag together. When we finally manage to get it in, we are both laughing at its weight. Indignant, Mom directs us to drop it in the kitchen.

"It's hot," Mom says, working the knob on the air conditioner. "Maybe we can go to Payne's Prairie or Ginnie Springs tomorrow, before you meet with the physicians?" she asks. My parents always do this. No matter where I am, they know more about the place than I do. Where every historical site is, how many Apaches were relocated there in the 1880s, and, of course, where they might find a red-bellied plover. Payne's Prairie is a large swamp south of

Gainesville. At the time, I hadn't heard of it. Or Ginnie Springs, where, according to my mother, crystal-clear blue water rises out of the limestone.

There's knocking and the front door swings open. "I want you to finally meet Terry," I say. Mom stops fiddling with the air conditioner and stares. Terry walks in. She is all smiles. There are warm introductions. We chat for a few minutes and then I go to my new hall closet to find towels, leaving Terry and my parents alone in the kitchen. I'm digging through bath towels when I hear Terry, her voice much louder than usual.

"OH MY GOD, is that what I THINK it is?"

"What?" I hear my mother say softly.

"Oh my God. OH MY GOD! DANIEL!" Terry yells.

What's wrong? I walk briskly back to the room, matching washcloths in my arms. I arrive in time to see my mother yank, and finally free, a massive, plastic Ziploc baggy from the Hoffa bag.

I know immediately that I have never seen this much marijuana crammed into such a small space. It must weigh a pound. The corners of the bag are splayed out and soon it's going to give birth to its contents.

Terry asks softly, "You didn't check that through . . ." She looks from my mother to me and then to my father.

"No one searched my bag," Mom says, flat. Then she sets the marijuana down in the middle of the kitchen table and walks over to the stove. She lifts my teapot and begins to fill it with water.

"We've got plenty more hanging in the attic if you need it. So, Terry . . . have you been to Ginnie Springs?"

Creedence Clearwater Biopsy

My regular checkup scans have been ambiguous lately. "There's a need for more information," the oncologist said. I'm in the surgery prep area. Another biopsy. They want to know if I've relapsed. I remember my other biopsies. Today they will go into my chest. I have headphones on and Creedence Clearwater Revival blares "Bad Moon Rising." It's not soothing music. It's passionate. Angry.

I had a biopsy six months ago. It was horrible. We suspected I'd relapsed, but the biopsy was negative and we were overjoyed. The news pleasantly eclipsed my memories of what happened during the surgery.

I'd been groggy but aware of the pain. My head was turned upward and away. My protests were feeble, as if the medications had anesthetized my language centers but left the pain. The surgeon refused to believe that I could feel him digging into my neck. There was no anesthesiologist assigned to the case and the nurse working with the surgeon only had access to weak painkillers.

I survey my little neighborhood. I am alone on a gurney in a preoperative waiting room. Long rows of gurneys are interrupted by a central nursing station where one nurse sits doing paperwork. Slow day, I muse. I was smart this time, I asked for an anesthesiologist. I long for her. If she's here, I'll be okay. She won't allow the surgeon to harm me. She came to my inpatient room yesterday. Instead of Dr. So-and-So, she introduced herself as Laura. She was in her late thirties. Pretty. Thin. Instead of a lab coat, the standard uniform of the attending physicians, she wore a housecoat, a smock. It had cartoon characters all over it. Bugs. Goofy. Roadrunner. She leaned against a wall and we talked. She asked about every surgery I could remember. But she also wanted to know about other things. The hospital food, my master's thesis, Terry's favorite movie.

In teaching hospitals there's a hierarchy. Medical student, intern, resident, fellow, attending. She is at the top of the tree. She knew her job well enough to relax. She seems to understand that healing takes more than technical competence.

Before she left she stepped up to me. Took my hand. Serious.

"I'm gonna be there during the surgery. I'm gonna take care of you." Matter-of-fact. No room for doubt. I felt my chest and shoulders relax, drop into the bed.

Two nurses appear and one chirps, "Moving time," and they wheel me into another room. I am heading for the surgery "on-deck" circle, as in baseball.

"This is silly," I say, propped up on my elbows. "I can walk. I haven't had any drugs or anything yet."

"Enjoy the ride," the chirpy one says.

After we arrive, a young man approaches my gurney. Clean-cut, he's dressed in operating room garb. Thin pants. A hair covering. Loose-fitting aqua shirt. A stethoscope around his neck. He introduces himself as the anesthesiologist. I watch the clean lines of his face. No stubble. I suspect he isn't old enough to need to shave. He asks for my arm and inspects the name tag bracelet. He looks from my wrist into my eyes as if he's a customs inspector and my passport has too many stamps. I consider telling him that I don't really need the biopsy, that I beat up another patient and took his name tag, but instead I just say "Yes?" and he says, "Oh, nothing." I wonder if he's contemplating how close we are in age.

He prepares to start an I.V. He gathers a needle and an alcohol wipe, and is diving for a vein when I interrupt him.

"You ought to use this one." I point to the crease inside my elbow where a thick blue vein resides.

"I need to use your hand," he says.

"No you don't," I insist. "It's the only good one—take what you can get."

He goes for my hand. Ouch. No luck. He has good technique but misses again. The rivulets of my hands have dried from the chemotherapy and sought shelter closer to the bone.

"Use this one," I say again, pointing at the thick blue river. He does. Score. I congratulate him. He does not appreciate this. He leaves. I should have asked about Laura.

I turn up the volume of the music—*Down on the corner / Out here on the street*—and close my eyes. What happened to her?

There must have been a switch. Maybe someone else's surgery went too long or she screwed up the schedule. I rub my neck where the first surgery was. For a moment it feels as though it still aches from the digging. That's silly, I realize. That pain is gone. I try some deep breathing. Calm myself down. I've read about people who could hypnotize themselves to not experience pain during surgery. Slow inhale. Slow exhale. A little better. But soon my thoughts return to Laura. *This young guy won't listen enough to help me with the pain. How will he know what to do? He wouldn't be here if he didn't know. That's not logical. They let me see patients after all, and much of the time I want to say, "Hmmm, you should really see a therapist." I'm alarmed that he didn't listen to me. He didn't trust me when I told him which vein to hit. And now I've antagonized him. Uh-oh.*

I can't get comfortable on this gurney. I've already slept eight hours and I'm not tired. My body needs to move around.

Two new nurses gather around me, short women wearing scrubs. They say something but I can't hear them, the music is too loud. I pull down the headphones. They are moving me to the O.R. It's time.

"Can we do a few laps around the hallways first? I'm starting to enjoy this gurney," I say, stalling. One giggles. No luck. I pull the headphones back up.

I study the ceiling tiles and vents as we move toward the O.R. We are through a doorway and I am wheeled under a large circular mirror with a light in the middle. It's bright. Someone says something and I'm moved, blankets and all, onto the operating table. My chest starts thumping. Someone tapes my finger to a line that runs to a pulse oximeter and I, and everyone, can hear my heart beating away in quick digital beeps. *Beepbeepbeep*. It's way too fast.

I look up and see the surgeon entering. He's already wearing a mask. Behind him, over his shoulder, I can see strands of blond hair peeking out from under a hair cover. Then the familiar housecoat. Donald and Bugs and Roadrunner.

The beeping slows. *Beep . . . beep . . . beep.*

Laura stands next to me. The others in the room are talking about something on the news, but she looks down into my eyes and takes my hand. The younger anesthesiologist, who I now realize is a resident, stands next to her. He looks out of place.

"In a minute I'm going to give you some medicines," Laura says. "I'm going to make sure you're comfortable, you don't need to worry. You can wear your headphones during the surgery if you'd like," she coos. I hear the beeps of my heart slowing as I put the headphones back on. I'm embarrassed by how much she soothes me. I can tell she's smiling at me because the creases near her eyes are wrinkled. She shows me the needle and I watch her push it into my I.V. I'm tapping my feet to "Down on the Corner" when the world drifts away.

Balance

The biopsy is over. The chest tube, designed to keep my lung inflated, is gone. They pulled it out with a one, two, three, OHMYGOD. I can't take deep breaths without stabbing pain, but I can breathe. And my energy isn't bad.

This time they tried to slice the beast from my chest. No success. I have a hazy memory of the surgeon telling Terry that scar tissue was everywhere, holding on to my lungs and my heart and my ribs. During the procedure a young surgeon nipped a lung and it deflated. But it's okay now. I can go home in a few days. The results of the biopsy will follow. Officially, we will know soon.

I don't tell Terry, but I know already. It's back. I know from the pain in my shoulder when I drink alcohol, the dots dancing across my vision again. I've played games with myself: Am I really in pain or is it just in my head? But I know. It's real pain. It's back.

We are in the hospital bathroom with the door closed. She watches me in the mirror. Her look is complex. She beckons but is passive, too. Pulls up her skirt. Wriggles. Her hair flows in and out of estuaries down the plane of her back. She is a portal back to life. In the next minutes I will leave behind the surgeries and statistics and blood pressure cuffs. In her I will swim back to burning leaves, long apple peels, and dripping summer roofs. This will not be lovemaking. It's too hungry. Desperate. Solemn.

She unbuttons her shirt and it hangs open, her hands on the sink, her back arched. She smiles at me in the bathroom mirror. I need her. I need this.

I hold on and we press together. She watches. And suddenly I can feel the strength in my biceps and thighs and I am young and powerful, vibrant and immortal. Slowly the world gathers together. When I was an adolescent I used to ride my ten-speed down a long hill near my childhood home and then, perfectly balanced, throw up my arms and look at the sky. And now, in this moment, I am at the bottom of the hill, it's autumn, and the air is crisp and I am strong. Unbeatable. I release and squeeze my eyes shut.

When I look Terry is smiling. As she uncouples she teases me in the mirror. "I told you nursing was superior to psychology; we offer many more holistic therapies than you guys." She pulls down her skirt and tries to straighten it. The nurses must be changing shifts now and soon one of them will be in my room. But I hold on, my arms wrapped around her breasts, my mouth buried in her neck. I can't bear to return to the bed. She smells of chamomile and I lean into her, drinking these last moments of balance.

Relapse

Delicate words floated in the white room. Pronounced in low tones. So practiced and somber. The fellow slowly adjusted his thin wire-rims.

". . . the specimens we recovered . . ."

I studied his accessories. A stethoscope. His beeper. Pens standing like trim soldiers in his pocket.

". . . still too early for full prognosis . . ."

He listed to and fro. As his weight shifted from foot to foot, I noticed he tended to lean a little longer on his left side. He's an uneven metronome.

". . . some success in the past . . ."

He cleared a dry throat.

". . . based on the staging . . ."

I looked up. The ceiling had a water spot in the middle of one of the perfect white squares.

". . . very serious . . ."

And out the window. It was overcast. I sipped juice through a straw. It made a slurping sound.

". . . profound abnormal growths."

I patted the bed near me, looking for an extra pillow. My back was sore. He stopped speaking and I looked at him.

His hand moved from his pocket to his chin. And back. Awkward. Then he removed his glasses and rubbed his eyes. I wondered if this was his first relapse proclamation. Maybe I remind him of a brother or a cousin. Giggles echoed down the long corridor outside my room.

Jodi and the Snow Leopard

A packet of information arrived at Vassar a few days after I was admitted to the University of Florida for graduate school. There was a list of apartment complexes including their varied amenities. I chose the cheapest of the group. Sunbay. From there I could walk to Shands Hospital, where I would spend most of the next five years seeing patients and taking classes.

Sunbay was twelve flat-roofed buildings, two community pools, and an office. The hallways smelled of curry and cigarettes. The apartments were inexpensive so they attracted graduate students, law students, and immigrants. People moved in from places as far away as the Philippines, Pakistan, and Ecuador, and as close as Jacksonville and Panama City. We swam together in the pool, shopped together at the Winn Dixie, and waited in the swampy concrete huts between the buildings for our laundry to finish.

When I returned from class I could see through the sliding glass doors into my neighbor's apartment. There were rugs and masks and other family heirlooms on the walls. My walls were barren, except for black-and-white photographs of my grandparents and great-grandparents, their hands awkward at their sides.

I started collecting things for my walls. I found a *Maltese Falcon* movie poster, university propaganda, and Ansel Adams photographs taken from a calendar. But my favorite find was a print from the New York Zoological Society, a watercolor of a snow leopard. It has blues and oranges, reds and greens. The leopard sits, its immense paws stretched forward. When I found it in the rack of animal posters, it stood out immediately. He looked right at me, relaxed and stress-free, the way I'd like to be.

As the work of graduate school classes piled up, I tried to remember the snow leopard. When the professor in our multivariate statistics class ordered us to calculate a factor analysis without a computer, I thought of the snow leopard. When we were warned that students were taking too long to get through the program, I thought of the snow leopard. When a few of the students dropped out, feeling too stressed to cope with the workload, I thought of the snow leopard.

The first patient I treated in graduate school was a girl named Jodi. My faculty sponsor, a gentle man, took me into his office in the middle of my first year. He sat me down. He explained that the program usually prohibited first-year graduate students from seeing patients. The program was designed to give clinical psychology trainees a strong foundation in theory and science before turning us loose on an unsuspecting population. But he was in a bind. There was an adolescent on the bone marrow transplant unit who needed help and might benefit from interacting with someone else who had also had cancer. He knew my history and was willing to circumvent the traditional program this one time. He didn't know we also had Hodgkin's disease in common.

He explained that Jodi hadn't spoken to anyone in over three weeks. There were concerns that she'd sunk into despair too deep for recovery. Or worse, that she'd suffered neurological damage from the chemotherapy or radiation. She wouldn't interact so it was difficult to tell.

The bone marrow transplant unit was on the fourth floor. Heavy double doors and a yellow sign warned entrants to wear gowns and coverings over shoes and hair. I pushed open the doors, interacted briefly with the pretty nursing supervisor, and tried to walk confidently down the long hall while I scanned the markered names on the doors. When I found the room, I paused at the door. My throat felt dry. I hummed and stepped inside. I tried to act as if I had worked in intensive care units for years. Her room had an anteroom with a sink, which had instructions posted over it about how to wash one's hands. It took a few moments to find the faucet switch on the floor. I pushed it with my foot and hot water gushed out, splashing my shirt. She watched from her bed.

When I turned and looked at her I noticed I.V. poles surrounding her like sentinels. Small square machines chirped and flashed green lights. The television was on, a fishing show. Not her choice, I guessed.

She was bald and swollen. It was clear that she was neurologically intact. She watched me like a caged cat who knew she couldn't escape, but also knew that I didn't belong. The walls were barren except for a few cards and photographs. Goofy cartoons with elephants and clowns.

"I'm impressed with what you've done with the place," I said. She raised an eyebrow with practiced cynicism. "New York

School of Design, right? Minimalism? How you doing?" She searched my hands for needles or maybe weapons. Finding none, she looked back at the television, uninterested. Not a peep.

I didn't know what psychologists did in these situations. Should I ask another question? Leave? I found a chair, sat down and watched fishing. A man was reeling a little fish onto his boat. He seemed to flex his biceps more than he needed to. After the third fish I stood up abruptly and left.

I started visiting Jodi whenever I had a break between classes. I'd come up to the unit, sit with her for five or ten minutes in silence. Day after day. I sat through cooking shows, soap operas, the weather, and real-estate infomercials. She didn't speak. Even after I told her about my illness. Nothing.

It was the water gun that changed everything. During a break between statistics and psychopathology I filled a bright yellow water gun with sterile water from a psychophysiology lab run by a friend.

I snuck the weapon onto the unit in a sealed sandwich bag under my shirt. Peeking into her room while she watched a soap opera, I took aim. The thin stream arched through the air and landed squarely. She blinked. Felt her face. Looked at the ceiling, curious. Then put her head down and reached for something. Her arm moved quickly and a crumpled ball of paper shot toward me from her bed, hitting me in the chin. She giggled. I was in.

Jodi started talking to me through parched lips, chapped like her entire intestinal system from total-body irradiation. She skeptically listened to my hopeful poems about her. Drank the orange Tylenol suspension I put into a shot glass to take down her fevers. Argued about the characters on her soap opera. And every now and then she even smiled.

Jodi was in the unit for more than sixty days.

Two months after she was released, I drove the five hours down to Venice Beach on Florida's west coast to see her. I stood with her parents in their dark house with its shag carpet and particleboard cabinets, talking while she slept. They told me she was sitting up at night, afraid to sleep. She'd nod off and then shake herself awake. They asked for my help.

When I saw her I had to steady myself. Time had played a devious trick, spinning weeks into decades. Her body had stiffened. She was hunched forward as if her neck was too weak to hold her head. She hugged me hard. Her body felt too warm and her eyes were cloudy and a little unfocused. We sat together and watched television again, like we had when we first met. Just before I left, when her parents were out of earshot, I whispered into her ear that she could rest now. Relax and stop fighting. It was okay. Anytime she wanted.

She died the next day.

Jodi's funeral was long-winded. A photo of her greeted entrants to the church. In the picture she had her own hair and was smiling, a self-conscious teenager with too much makeup and puffy hair. We went to her house after the ceremony. There were platters of hors d'oeuvres in every corner — deviled eggs, pâté, and miniature hot dogs. Teenagers milled about. When we arrived her mother cut through a small group, took my hand and took me into Jodi's bedroom. She gave me a bag of stuffed animals and a few Madonna cassettes, telling me, "She wanted you to take these." Then she went to her closet and pulled out the yellow water gun. "And this."

Six months later my relapse was diagnosed. My first instinct was to flee the medical system. I knew that a bone marrow transplant would be the next treatment on the menu and I couldn't shake Jodi's demise. I saw her in my mind whenever I thought about my options. In the image she was hunched toward me, her shoulders and neck stiff with disease, her eyes cloudy.

I knew that oncologists frequently offered aggressive treatments to patients even when the odds were grim and I'd never seen a patient with Hodgkin's disease survive a transplant. I knew there were some who had, but I'd never met one.

A few nights after the relapse diagnosis I had a dream. I've never paid much attention to the nightly entertainment sweeping across the stage of my mind. Instead, I prefer to think of dreams as random stories. But this dream felt different.

I was trudging upward through a jagged winter blanket of snow and rock. I wore a heavy backpack and the air was crisp and thin. The sky was a dark blue. There were no trees. Just rock. High above, a massive world of jutting angles threatened. Black. Gray. White. My fingers and toes were numb. The grade grew harsh and I pulled for air. *If I just rest for a second, I can catch my breath.* I stopped, doubled over for a few moments, and drank in the air. When I started walking again my foot missed its target and my balance was suddenly precarious. *Will I fall?* I froze. Afraid to go up. Afraid to go down. Trepidation swirled in my belly.

A trickle of white descended and gathered around my numb toes. I looked up the mountain. There was a crack from above, a metal-striking-metal sound. *Avalanche?* My eyes went wide. I inhaled quickly. A blind gasping terror.

Then, from nowhere, a beast dropped in front of me. Its paws slapped at the snow and ice. Its fur was bright. Purples and blues and yellows and reds and greens spotted its shoulders, neck and face. Corded powerful limbs flexed beneath the fur. It turned toward me. Its eyes bored into mine. Familiar. Resilient, seasoned veteran's eyes. I gasped and leaned backward, almost falling.

"Drop your pack," the snow leopard boomed, its voice low and commanding. "Climb aboard my back. I will carry you."

I didn't move.

"NOW!" he demanded. I awkwardly removed the pack, stepped, one foot, then another, toward the beast. He was unflinching.

Then I was on his back and we were bounding upward, over rock and snow and ice, and then flying, lifting quickly, and the mountain receded beneath my feet and the air was cool and gentle and effortless and the world was the brightest blue.

When I awoke I went into the bathroom to pee. On my way back to bed I saw the poster. It looked different. The snow leopard looked resolute. Fierce. Ready.

When I was admitted to the bone marrow transplant unit I was assigned Jodi's old room. I brought in the print and tacked it to the wall.

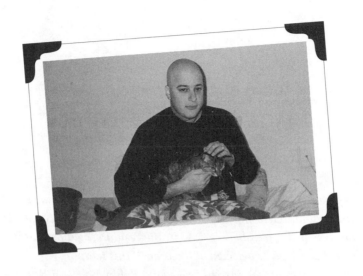

Part Three

Bone Marrow Transplant

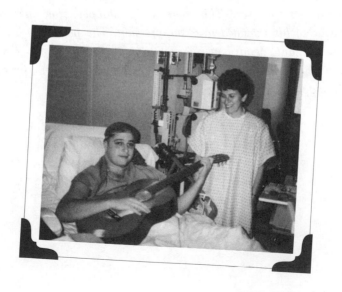

Dictated Chart Note

7/90

The patient underwent nodal biopsy. Pathology confirmed recurrent nodular sclerosing Hodgkin's disease. Further CT scan evaluation revealed a possible increase in the residual mediastinal mass. No other disease is detected at the time of this relapse.

The patient was referred and evaluated by Dr. Saul Rosenberg at Stanford University. Dr. Rosenberg recommended the patient undergo six cycles of ABVD chemotherapy followed by an autologous bone marrow transplant. The patient was referred back here to the University of Florida for treatment. He underwent one cycle of ABVD but was unable to tolerate this therapy due to poor hematopoetic recovery. This therapy was stopped after one cycle because of his extended myelosuppression. The patient will now receive an autologous bone marrow transplant. The probability of surviving transplant is 75%, the 5 year survival rate, given his current relapse, is at least 40%.

CHARLES ERIC SCHULMAN, M.D.
Shands Hospital at the University of Florida

Unfriends

Jack and I immediately recognized that we were different breeds. He was Southern, Catholic, conservative, and an excellent sales-man. He had short-cropped hair that was carefully groomed. I am Northern, Jewish, slightly to the left of Lenin, and artsy. When we met, I had graduate student–length hair and an earring.

The trouble started after his first Jewish joke. It was the first time I'd heard a Jewish joke told by a non-Jew in which the pro-tagonist fit the stereotype (Jews are greedy, manipulative, etc.) perfectly. The joke was something about a dead Jewish man try-ing to buy his way into heaven despite having a checkered past. All the Jewish jokes I'd heard had been told by Jews making fun of the stereotype. He knew I was Jewish. And yet the stereotype was so much a part of his life that he wasn't even embarrassed. He laughed heartily and reached out and tapped my shoulder playfully. He even seemed mildly annoyed when my facial fea-tures froze. Our relationship went downhill from there.

I figured Jack enjoyed hunting, golf, and meat that bled when you pushed a fork into it. I suspected he went to church every Sunday more because his wife wanted him to than out of personal conviction. I knew he would tolerate fatherhood but never take to it with vigor. He was a man's man. A beer drinker who never thought much about what he saw on the news. I put him in a mental box with Archie Bunker; the kids at college who enjoyed blasting Van Halen while breaking dorm furniture; Mike Stanavicius, the racist wrestling captain; and Richie Shulik, who, when I was six, drew a swastika and gave it to me to see how I would react. I taped up the box and put it away, hoping it would be a while before I needed to put someone else in there.

When we spent time together (Terry and his wife were close friends) I overtly feigned interest in him while subtly digging at him with offbeat comments about his education, his hobbies, and his interests. Later, alone with Terry, I wondered aloud how his wife found him interesting.

When Jack gave up his job to take care of their first baby I was shocked. He changed diapers, warmed frozen breast milk, and rocked the baby back to sleep at four A.M. He did laundry, cooked dinner, and vacuumed the living room. He pushed a shopping cart at midday and evaluated the grapefruit while keeping one ear open for his baby's cries. It confused me, but I figured he wasn't quite the salesman he said he was and had no other options.

When they found cancer in my body again, word spread like a dusty Western fire through our friendships. I learned later that it was eleven at night when Jack heard the news. His wife had just returned, exhausted, from the evening shift at the hospital. Jack fed his wife her dinner, did the dishes, and tucked her into bed. He got the car seat, packed up his baby, and drove to church. He walked down the dark aisles of the church carrying his sleeping son, got down on his knees, and prayed to his God for me.

Time

Bone marrow transplant is a misnomer. I had an autologous bone marrow transplant, meaning that I donated bone marrow to myself. Chemotherapy killed rapidly dividing cells, not discriminating between those healthy and diseased. Bone marrow is the factory that produces cells. I could take otherwise lethal doses of chemotherapy because I would receive my own, unmarred, bone marrow back afterward. Once bone marrow arrives back home it goes right to work, like a platoon of army engineers back from R&R. After six straight days of receiving megadoses of chemotherapy I was transplanted.

I was transplanted in June. In Gainesville, summers are wet, humid, and alive. Insects large enough to steal books out of your hands command the heavy air. At four in the afternoon, virtually every day, the sky opens up and soaks everything. As quickly as the storms come they're gone. Thin streams of water swirl on hot pavement, steam rises, and shirts stick to hot bodies. But inside my room on the BMTU it was a steady seventy-two degrees with a light breeze from the northeast.

Before the transplant I had many tests. Scales, scanners, scalpels. Professionals peeked into every orifice. They also installed a central line, three plastic tubes taped unceremoniously to my belly. It ran directly into my femoral vein just west of my groin. The tubes allowed infusions of chemotherapy and blood draws without my constantly being stuck with needles. The central line gradually became part of my landscape, bridging the distance between the not-me and the me. I played with it as if it were an earlobe or a familiar ring.

Because transplant patients are dangerously immune-compromised, there were strict rules in the room. I was forbidden from touching anything that had not been gassed or Cloroxed first. I couldn't touch the floor with bare feet. I used a commode in the middle of the room to avoid moving out of air control. During one early conversation with a doctor, I jokingly threatened to kill myself by throwing myself, naked, onto the floor. He did not think it was funny.

The transplant started with six days of high-dosage chemotherapy. Cytoxan and VP-16. Two days of rest. Then I received my own bone marrow back. The symptoms started quickly. Before the transplant, in other treatments, I'd always had brief infusions and then at least a week to recover. Never six days in a row. At the end of the first, long, dizzying day of chemotherapy, a montage of darkness and light, nausea and fatigue, I said to Terry, "This has been a long day."

"Sweetheart," she whispered. "It's the fourth day."

Bird Counts

For bird people, birds are mysterious creatures that grace our lives with their presence. For them the arch of an outstretched wing or the chirp of an amorous suitor quickens the heartbeat and stirs the soul. True bird people, I learned as I grew up, spend hours studying bird maps. They balance precariously on ladders to reach ideally located feeders. They traipse through marsh and swamp when the sun is still waking up. Some even install heaters to prevent birdbaths from freezing over. Due to some unnatural genetic accident I was not born a bird person. My parents, on the other hand, entered life by pecking themselves out of enormous eggs.

Throughout my life I've listened to them discuss the intricacies of mating, the mysteries of migration and the connections between finches and pterodactyls. As long as I can remember, my mother has kept her North American bird book near her at all times. She keeps it in an aging backpack along with an army-issue pair of binoculars equipped with night vision and heat detection. I remember one conversation that took place in our household when I was twelve. It was reenacted in various forms at highway rest stops, in restaurants, and near the mall.

My mother rushed to the dining-room window of our suburban Connecticut home and sang, "Oh, look, honey, a Crested Auklet!"

My father flung away his crossword puzzle and raced to the window, knocking over a chair in the process. "Where, where?!" he pleaded, looking eagerly into the backyard. She stretched a finger toward a birdfeeder, but then it drooped. "Oh, darn. He's gone."

"Did you say Crested Auklet?" he asked, incredulous.

"Well, it could have been a Whiskered Auklet, but they're rare."

He fingered through the bird book. "Hmmm." Skeptical. "It says here Crested Auklets are only seen on the Aleutian or Shumagin Islands off Alaska."

My mother responded, "Yeah, honey, that's why I'm so surprised. How exciting. I only feel bad because you didn't get to see it." She then carefully wrote the date of the sighting next to the picture of the bird in her book: *Crested Auklet, dining room window, August 14, 1978.*

My parents rented an apartment to be near me during my bone marrow transplant. After six days of chemotherapy I got my bone marrow back and we started waiting. During this period all of my blood counts dropped like hail. My white counts and platelets dropped to zero. We all knew this was dangerous. I was vulnerable to infections. The sooner my counts climbed, the faster I'd be allowed to go home.

The medical team kept track of my counts on a lined page tacked to the wall. A few days after the transplant my parents visited.

Mom greeted me. "You look great. Your counts are improving, aren't they?"

Behind her, my father surveyed the chart. Squinted at it.

"Says here his counts are zero," my father reported.

Mom studied me. "He looks good to me. He's got more color, he's more alert, and his skin tone isn't so blotchy. Yup. That chart's wrong. His counts are improving, I can tell."

My father looked at me. "Maybe," he said, then he came closer and stood next to her. "I guess he does look a little less blotchy."

"You'll be out of here before you know it," Mom declared.

I was skeptical, but the next day my counts were significantly better. And even better the next, as she continued to predict.

And to this day, I'm sure that somewhere, in a familiar backyard in northern Connecticut, there's an Alaskan Crested Auklet, and, by now, a whole extended family, enjoying their new home.

David

I awoke to the knock, curled into my bed. The drone of the airflow machines reminded me where I was. Tubes ventured from under my blankets out into whirring machines. David, my brother, steadied himself to look in on me for the first time. I had no energy to think about how he might respond. There was nothing I could do to protect him. He would have to take care of himself this time.

My brother has always been eccentric. When he was eleven he wore a watch on each wrist. When I asked him why he needed two watches he held up his right hand, sober, and waved it gently. "This one tells accurate time," he told me, and he lifted up his left hand and shook it: "This one fits." He was serious.

When we were nine and six we created an elaborate world that we played in for the next four years. In it we were orphans who lived in an underground city. We had escaped an orphanage and bonded together with other boys to form our own society. Other groups of boys had done similar things and we were at war with them, and with the original orphanage, who had hired goons to track us down and bring us back. At flea markets we purchased old, nonworking electronic equipment and then took some toys and strung the lot together with old stereo wire in our playroom, making a command center. There were old phones, keyboards, adding machines, and even a battleship game. On large pads of paper we drew up architectural diagrams that showed the entire city and posted them on the wall. We had bowling alleys, arcades, meeting rooms, and many alternatives for eating, including a peanut-butter-and-jelly stand that my brother insisted on.

When we were separated for camp or when David went on week-long field trips we wrote letters to each other, signing off with our code names. When we were in the car or after school, we'd plan for an attack, or hide in the woods near our house, evading capture. Once we invited a neighborhood kid to join us, but it just didn't work. He didn't understand our culture. We spent most of our time planning and working out strategies. Only a little of the time was spent in combat. The friend kept wanting to go outside and fight the bad guys.

Years later, when I started wrestling, I'd practice on David. I'd push all the living-room furniture against the couch and stand him up facing me. But as soon as I leaned into him to do a move involving at least three of his extremities he'd drop to the floor, close his eyes, roll over on his back and pretend to be dead. I think he hoped I would respond like the bears we'd read about in *National Geographic*. Perhaps I would just sniff at him and go away. I didn't. I practiced moves called wizard, and popcorn, and grapevine, and switch, and quarter nelson, and chicken wing.

If I was too rough and our parents were in the house, he would cry out in an abrasive singsong, "Dannnnnyyyyy," and my mother, cued, would scream that I should stop abusing my brother.

Occasionally David and I would be quietly reading alone and he would suddenly grin at me, almost giggling, his eyes scrunched up. "Don't you dare," I'd threaten. But out would come that piercing wail, "Dannnnnnyyyyy," and our mother would yell at me to leave my poor brother alone.

David left London after his junior year abroad, but instead of traveling around Europe as he'd planned, he moved in with my parents in Gainesville. All of them shared a two-bedroom apartment for the summer so they could be near me during my transplant.

Initially my parents were irritated that David didn't find work. "You need to earn some money while you're here," they told him. "This isn't vacation." So during the days he worked making pizzas or playing piano at the Holiday Inn and visited me in the evenings. His girlfriend was far away and he longed for her. As my parents grew obsessed with my cell counts, my sleep and variations in the clarity of my thinking, David was only noticed when his living habits conflicted with theirs. He didn't keep his room clean. He borrowed my car and had a fender bender in a parking lot that wasn't his fault. We were furious with him. "Can't you stay out of trouble?"

When I was discharged from the unit David made snide comments to me at every opportunity. He harassed me as never before. "God, Dan, you are ugly. What did they do to you in there?" When I took a few moments longer to get up stairs: "Damn, you're slow." And worse: "You look scary. . . ." And he jabbed a finger into my chest. Angry.

When the transplant team cleared me for swimming, my brother and I drove to Ginnie Springs. We were treading water together when David poked toward my face. "Look at you, flabby man." I grabbed him suddenly. I was afraid for a moment that I wouldn't have enough strength, but my hands clamped reliably. We descended ten ear-popping feet, and I twisted him so I was behind him. This was nothing new. David and I have wrestled in water since we were children. Despite the transplant and weakness I still had strong lung volume. Years of living with no lung capacity, my lungs squeezed by the grapefruit-sized tumor, had accustomed me to the faint tickles of oxygen deprivation. I'd learned to tolerate the dark heaviness of mental slowing.

I held him hard against me and we sat together on the bottom. I could hear my heart slowing in my ears and could see his long hair drifting over both of us. Eventually I let him go, seconds later than he expected. We ascended quickly. After we took our first, deep, luxurious gasps, I kicked away from him expecting a physical response. When I looked back I saw a familiar warmth in his eyes.

"Dannnyyyyyyyyyyyyy," he sang playfully.

Dirty Pencils

During the transplant, my head went fuzzy. It was three weeks before I was thinking clearly again. I was bald and weak. The central line ran from my body to a number of I.V. poles hovering nearby. A urinal was clipped to the side of the bed so I didn't have to get up to pee, and I needed help to get to the commode. My intestinal tract was sloughing itself off and the distinguishing features of my face had receded beneath prednisone flab. I now had no privacy and little control of my environment.

It was cool in the room (baldness makes the world considerably colder), but I felt warm under the blankets. I found the pencil and pad I'd stashed in a bedside table. Words were going to organize my experience and liberate me for a few moments from my struggle. For some people, talking to a friend releases internal demons. For me, writing of my experiences brushes a healing balm of perspective on them. I understand the why and how of things after I write them down. I understand what I want and what I don't want.

I started to write, but my unpracticed hand lost the pencil and it tumbled, end over end, bouncing onto the floor. I remembered the rules. Once it hit the floor I was forbidden from touching it. I leaned over the bed and stared at the pencil.

I imagined standing in front of St. Peter. Him in flowing white robes, surveying a clipboard, saying, "Well, everything looks as if it's in order: I just have one last question. How'd you die?" Then me mumbling, "Er, I uh, I, I touched a pencil . . ." and him slowly shaking his head.

I reached down to get it. As my arm descended I felt my thigh push against something and then I was wet; I'd spilled my urinal.

The blanket quickly soaked through. Suddenly I was drenched in my own cold piss and the stench filled the small room; I felt it on my calves and thighs, my loins and belly.

I felt as if a heavy, suffocating curtain had been dropped on me. In a heartbeat I went from feeling empowered and optimistic to thoroughly dehumanized. I sat there for a long time. I could have hit the call light for nursing help but didn't.

I felt frozen, weary, beaten down. Tired of fighting. I saw myself standing on a ledge, high over a void. It was too deep to see the bottom and I knew it could suck away sound and light. I felt isolated and had no voice. Just a dying, bloated body.

I still didn't move.

Eventually a nurse, Erica, came into the room. She mentioned something about the weather, and then, with a few efficient movements I was clean, had dry, warm blankets, a soft touch on the arm, and a fresh pencil . . . and she was gone. In the flap of a wing I was brought back. Restored.

I didn't thank her right then for the touch of her fingers on my arm, for her casual, matter-of-fact appraisal, or for the perspective she brought into the room. I wasn't oriented enough to attach words to my experience.

With her practiced, gentle style, movements she made hundreds of times a day, she rehumanized me. I'm certain the number of times in my life I'll move, so quickly, between such radical extremes will be counted on one hand. But when I went back to thank her weeks later, she had no memory of the event. She politely acknowledged my thanks and smiled, awkward, looking away, not understanding the passion behind my praise.

Water Medicine

I'd seen Jodi's experience. The machines hovering around her as she grew weaker. The plastic toilet in the middle of the room. The silent television and fishing shows. The smell of antiseptic permeating the airless room. The blank gray walls.

During social psychology class my freshman year of college, Dr. Cornelius had shown us slides of different buildings and asked for our impressions. He taught us that buildings surrounded by weeds and cracked pavement are more frequently spray-painted with graffiti, workers in rooms with windows and plants concentrate better, and harpists in intensive care units can soothe and strengthen heartbeats.

I thought carefully about the things I wanted to bring with me onto the unit. I started with the walls. I put up the snow leopard print. I brought in an erotic print of a woman, the curves of her waist and ribs peeking from beneath silk. And cards from wellwishers to remind me of friends and family.

I brought in a remote-controlled light socket and switch, a red light bulb and plenty of extension cord. I wired the apparatus over the window of the door so that from my bed I could turn on a red light to warn incoming professionals and visitors that I wanted privacy — time to sit on the commode, throw up, or just be alone.

I brought in a simple stereo and music for every mood. Bach, Mozart, Vivaldi. Simon and Garfunkel, James Taylor, Led Zeppelin, Queen, Pink Floyd.

I spoke to the owner of Gainesville Health and Fitness, my health club. A few days into the transplant two burly men appeared pushing a professional exercise bike replete with flashing lights and digital readouts.

I brought in goofy things. A battery-operated water gun. A Groucho Marx nose and glasses.

I brought in books and magazines. Adventures and erotica, humor and drama.

I brought in my trusty notebook and writing materials.

A VCR. Movies.

In concert these changes altered the social landscape of the room. It became a real person's room. My room. Unlike Jodi's room, the same physical space, it was no longer anonymous, owned by the professionals who inhabit the unit. It belonged to me. The red light, in particular, altered the power structure because it gave me, a mere patient, some control over who entered the room when I was awake. In exchange, I agreed not to turn on the light when I was sleeping so the staff could get work done: change dressings, dispense medications, and clean.

As I grew sicker I moved my implements of control closer. Tissue boxes, urinals, receptacles. The remote for the privacy light, VCR, and stereo. I pulled up an additional food tray and stacked my other diversions. Books, notebook, and toys. I kept them all organized and within arm's reach.

One Monday morning a team of physicians I hadn't met appeared in my room. There were three of them. Each was dressed crisply — white shirt, conservative tie, lab coat. They had a legitimate, official air about them, like pilots or attorneys. An older one, his hairline receding into gelled gray, motioned to a younger one. The younger one started, "This is a twenty-three-year-old single Caucasian male who underwent an autologous bone marrow transplant eleven days ago for stage IIb relapsed Hodgkin's with bulky nodular sclerosing disease whose conditioning regimen included high-dose Cytoxan and VP-16 and . . ."

He was looking right at me but talking to the others. Gesturing. It reminded me of how my art history professor used to talk at the screen, his entire hand jabbing into it like a canoe paddle. "Notice the ionic column work" or "Tintoretto's brush stoke here is particularly notable."

I studied their faces. They were somber. Professional. Removed. The younger one, who was talking, began describing my blood counts.

Clearing my throat, I managed to raise a voice, an achievement given the potholed state on the inside of my mouth. "Excuse me," I muttered. "Who are you?" My voice sounded early-morning low and uneven.

The older one, the attending physician, looked from me to the younger one, who appeared to be about twenty-five, a resident, I guessed. Then the older one tipped his head back quickly, a slight gesture, but definite. He was telling the resident to continue. The younger one looked from his teacher to me and then back. He continued, "His CBC for today obviously isn't back yet, but yesterday—"

"Excuse me?" I asked again. Was there something wrong with my voice? Maybe he couldn't hear me? "Who are you guys?" I asked. Louder.

The attending physician scrunched up his forehead. Then he brought out his hand from a pocket and held it up to me. I could see his raised fingers. He was giving me the crossing guard's stop sign! SILENCE! the hand said. Then the hand turned, palm open, knuckles down, toward the resident. Go, the hand said to him.

"As I said . . ." continued the resident.

I felt the room slipping from me. Now it was his. With a simple gesture he had reclaimed the space. Made it his. But I needed it more. Deserved it more.

"Who are you guys?" I asked again, still louder, despite the hand. I felt a twinge of conditioned guilt. Crossing when the guard said "Stop." But I did have a voice. It was even clear and audible.

He'd anticipated me. With the first sounds of my voice his hand shot up again and extended until it was as far away from his shoulder as it could get. An eyebrow raised. His lips tightened. STOP.

I felt something. Some forgotten chord resonated, deep, in my chest. Like when I was sixteen and the supermarket manager leaned into me and told me I hadn't been working hard enough to deserve my break, and like when I was twelve and the bully grabbed my bike and told me it was his now.

As the resident continued, I reached for my trusty friend. . . .

I was initially attracted to the box because of the packaging. The large box was emblazoned with bold black letters, 30 FOOT SOAKER. It showed a boy in obvious terror running for cover in the far distance. At the top of the box, a finger squeezed the trigger of a device that looked to be the ultimate in water weaponry: fake chrome barrel, black trigger, orange tubes wrapped around the handle.

The resident persisted, "So, in summary, this is a twenty-three-year-old Caucasian male with—AN UZI!"

In retrospect, I'm not sure I fully appreciated the dramatic volume of water that would erupt from the nozzle. It's immaterial now. I remember reaching for the weapon and pulling it up quickly. Squeezing the plastic trigger. I remember a thick stream of pulsing water shooting out of the nozzle.

The rest is something of a blur. I think there were hands raised in defense and a few sputtered utterances of surprise. I'm pretty sure I remember seeing a wad of gray hair drooping over a wet forehead. The next thing I definitely remember, I was alone in the room, thinking, Wow, those guys could really move.

I anticipated a guilty pang for my adolescent behavior but none materialized. Instead I felt liberated. I even got out of bed for the first time in a few weeks, slowly moved across the floor, and straightened the snow leopard print.

A few days later a combed young head peeked into my room. The younger one. He said he'd read the sign on the door about the light, and since it wasn't on . . . was this a good time? He stepped in, washed his hands in the anteroom, and asked if he could sit down. "Sure," I told him.

He started by introducing himself by his first name. Joshua. He admired the art on the wall and commented on the movie I'd been watching, *The Maltese Falcon*. He even did a brief Peter Lorre impersonation.

He looked different than I'd remembered, then I realized he wasn't wearing his lab coat. He had the tie but his collar was ruffled and I could see stubble along his neck where his shaver had missed. He started asking questions, simple at first, and then more probing. Was I able to eat? Had I used the bike? And how was my family doing? After I answered, tentative at first, he asked others. How was I keeping my spirits up? What was the prognosis for relapsed Hodgkin's disease? He listened. Seemed genuinely interested. He shared how hard his residency was, how little sleep he was getting, and how his attending physician had a fondness for medical trivia. I found myself telling him things. How I tried to pass the time on the unit. My fear of infections.

We didn't talk about the water gun; it was as if it hadn't happened. We were two people meeting each other for the first time. Eventually he asked permission to see a rash on my leg, the real reason for the initial visit. As he looked at it he explained why it could have been infectious, why his team had been called, and told me about the ointment he wanted the nurses to put on it. Then we shook hands, he patted me on the shoulder, and was gone.

The rash cleared up quickly, but to this day I'm not sure which medicine was more effective, the ointment or the water.

Basketball Dreams

During the summer before graduate school Chuck, Jay, Eric and I spent our time working odd jobs in Cambridge, swimming in Walden Pond, carousing at the Pour House, and playing speed chess in Harvard Square. But more than anything else, we played basketball. Chuck is short, quick, and has a strong outside jump shot. He's unstoppable when hot. A usually funny and gentle guy, his personality changes when he's on the court to loud and street-wise. Eric is the tallest of the group. He's wiry and strong. Unmovable beneath the basket. Jay is the shortest of the group but the most athletic. He moves at full speed with the ball, spinning, arching, leaping.

I have no such talent. Despite years on the court—dribbling drills, passing practice, jump shots—I remain pathetic. Imagine trying to dribble a deflated beach ball. That's me with a basketball. Nor can I rebound, shoot, or pass well. I've got no vertical leap and no natural grace. I can't even taunt with conviction.

We played two on two that summer. We switched the teams frequently. I'd be paired with each of them. Regardless of which of the poor souls found me on his side, he'd be encouraging.

"If you have the open shot, take it. You the man!" Chuck pointed at me.

"Stick 'em, Danny, you can do it!" Eric would yell.

"You the money man, baby!" Jay would howl.

I'd been on the bone marrow transplant unit for two weeks, despondent and disoriented, when someone knocked on my door. A tall head hovered in the doorway. Eric. I learned later that he'd left Duke's summer session and flown to New York and then Boston. Then he circled back and flew to Gainesville. He told his physics professors there was something he had to do.

He stepped into my room carrying a five-foot basketball hoop complete with backboard and Nerf basketball. He'd checked it through Delta Airlines. Written across the backboard were markered phrases written in different hands.

You the man! and *Stick 'em Danny!* and *You the money man, baby!*

Summertime

I'm fourteen days into the transplant and this morning the airflow machine sounds remind me of rain on a tin roof in the summer. Shadows flutter on the wall, hovering like osprey. The plastic bag hanging on the I.V. pole looks like a conch, slick and curled, shiny, my sea trumpet. The overhead lights are Chinese lanterns strung across my sail, and the central line is a seaweed loincloth. Then all the images come together: This bed is a flat-bottom boat, the privacy curtain my sail, and I'm a brave salt river king, following the unpredictable flat water toward some romantic destiny.

My mind does strange things in here. I have vivid visions, some fantasy and some memory, all playing out as if they're happening now. I don't think they are ICU psychosis, the craziness that visits people who are sleep deprived and denied stimulation. I'm sleeping quite a bit and there's plenty of stimulation. I think I just have a strange, overactive imagination.

This morning, before the image of the river, when it was still dark outside but I was awake, I felt as if I was in the New Jersey parks of my earliest childhood. Summertime. The smells of cigars, cut grass, and barbecue, the shouts of soccer players, some in shorts and some in work clothes, running through the humidity. I could even see the pigeons, moving like old men, bobbing as they walked.

Then, as the sun came up, the shadows on the ceiling reminded me of the fish at the New England aquarium. I remembered the *thwuck* sound of a little hand patting thick glass, my hand, and hypnotically watching the mindless multicolored dancers darting and lollygagging, close and then disappearing.

Later, when it was quiet, I was back down in the Vassar library stacks. Floors below the massive stained-glass window, and the long rows of cherry-oak tables, there's a small room filled with old philosophy and psychology books. Near the low ceiling there are short windows that let in dusty light up at ground level. During my summer at Vassar, when I was doing research between chemotherapy hits, it was a quiet sanctuary. I loved the books, their weight and the slick heavy paper. The lithograph inscriptions and elegant fonts. The feel of old parchment and wisdom printed in heavy inks. I'm there at an old wooden desk, surrounded by Pascal and Spinoza, William James and John Watson.

Is my life passing before my eyes or are these the result of all the opiates I've ingested? *The scenes were all set in the summer.* Summers that were, summers that could be. And I feel it, my body longs for the splash of pools and lakes. For fried food and wet towels, sunscreen and mosquito repellent. Sand-filled boat shoes and bathing suit drawstrings. But instead I'm in here, where it's a steady seventy-two degrees.

Summerless.

Clams and Ballet

Every summer we took a family vacation. We always went by car, usually pulling the pop-up trailer. We never had much money, so the vacations were budgeted carefully. One year we drove from Hartford to the Colorado Rockies, another year to Orlando, and a few times up to Nova Scotia. In the backseat, David and I played Dice Baseball, a game my father invented in which dice rolls represent different batting outcomes. Dice Baseball was the perfect intersection of math and baseball, two of my father's favorite things. Using his game, we could pit the '75 Red Sox, our favorite team, against my father's '69 Mets or the old Brooklyn Dodgers. I'd roll for each of our players and David or Mom would roll for Dad. My brother and I never complained that the Mets beat our Red Sox every time we played. One of Dad's hitters would take Luis Tiant deep and Dad would shake his head, looking at us in the rearview mirror: "You guys give up yet?"

Aside from the frequent stops to look at the birds Mom hallucinated seeing or hearing, we enjoyed the drives and were good car travelers. One year, mostly because of car troubles involving a liquid my father referred to as sludge, we just went to the Maine shore. We had to stop a few times to let Dad peer under the hood and make diagnostic grunts, but other than some mysterious smoke it was an uneventful drive. When we arrived at the campground, it took my parents, neither of whom is graced with mechanical prowess, about forty minutes to back the trailer into the site and "pop it up." As a child it appeared to me that the act of raising the trailer required a minimum of one yelling argument.

While they argued David and I explored the campground. Then we competed for who would be the first to swing open the little plastic door of the trailer and climb in, like astronauts entering a deserted space pod. The trailer had a small pull-out kitchen and cardboard cabinets under three fold-out beds. I liked it. It smelled of campfires, canvas and vacation.

The next morning Mom and I were the first ones up. She suggested we go clamming, so off we walked to the beach. When we got there we waited for the tide to empty out of a cove. When it was far enough out we rolled up our pants and took off our shoes. Mom gave me a bucket and a spade. "Now you're a certified clam hunter," she said. She pulled a wide-brimmed straw hat over her head and gave me my Red Sox cap. We ventured out into the mud and foam. We traipsed until my calves were covered with mud. Then she stopped me. "Look," she said, and pointed. There were crabs, spiral-colored mollusks, and hundreds of other little critters making their lives in the thin film of cold salt water and sand.

Mom directed my gaze to bubbles rising from small holes. "Prepare for infiltration," she announced. Then her hand darted into the mud, down through the bubbles, and magically pulled out a clam the size of her hand. She washed it off in her bucket, turned it over, and showed me its neck and the membrane holding the shell together.

"You want to eat it now?" she offered, holding it up to my face. "Just kidding." She laughed at me. She put the clam in my bucket.

Hours later, when the tide started in and my face felt hot and salty, we retreated. I hopped at the edge of the ocean with a towel and sandals, awkwardly trying to remove the sand from my feet, and my mother told me I had good balance. Maybe someday I would dance like Baryshnikov.

That night, back at the campsite, we put all the clams in a large pot and boiled them over an open fire. It was a dark night, with far more stars than I was used to. Ordered to find more kindling, I wandered away from the site and got lost. My faint flashlight threw a modest circle of orange light on trees and wood chips. I walked faster and faster through the woods and other people's campsites wondering where my family was. A fantasy flashed through my mind, of my family packing up, quickly pulling down the pop-up trailer and jumping into the car.

Eventually, through no skill of my own, I found the fading light of our fire, my mother's face illuminated near the clam pot, my father and brother stripping branches. I felt relief in my arms and neck, like being wrapped in a warm blanket after being outside on a cold night.

During my bone marrow transplant Mom and Dad visited frequently. Sometimes too frequently and we fought. I remember one morning when Mom had been hovering around me, a constant annoying presence. It culminated when she opened a bag of chips for me and I yelled at her, infuriated, "I can do that for myself!" She welled up, indignant, and threw the chips on the bed and quickly left the room. I put the chips on a side table and curled up, falling asleep.

A dream unfolded. I was back in those dark campsites, fumbling over wood chips and rocks, tent cords and coolers. I scrambled from site to site, finding scraps of fabric from my brother's denim jacket, dice from our game, and broken clam shells.

I woke up with remnants of the dream still lingering, the

smell of wood chips and campfire. Mom was nearby, she was back, sitting near my bed, putting together a puzzle. And suddenly I felt that relief in my arms and neck, the comfort of being with someone who always saw potential for ballet in my awkwardness and could always help me find nourishment, even in the sand.

Parole

Greenhaven has tall gray walls that interrupt the oak, maple, and sycamore surrounding it. If you weren't looking for the prison, you wouldn't find it. It's on a single-lane road in the middle of farm country, about ninety minutes north of New York City. The first time I worked there I was surprised. Not by its immense size, but by the quiet. Behind the walls there were thousands of men working and living. But outside there was no trace of them. Just a vast, silent parking lot scattered with vehicles.

Inside, I stood in a quiet, orderly line, awaiting my turn at the metal detector. When it was my turn, I untied my high-tops and handed them to a burly female sergeant who searched them. Then I signed in. Someone stamped my hand with invisible ink. From there I began my trek through steel doors and long echoing corridors.

We followed dull yellow lines painted on the concrete floors. "Stay to the right of the yellow and you'll be just fine," my escort said. The inmates we encountered along the route walked angled so they could see both in front and behind them. They wore drab workshirts and gray institutional pants. Their hairstyles were dated—Afros, "pork chop" sideburns, and Jheri curls. Long mustaches.

Once at the Prerelease Center, I signed in again and stepped into the program offices, two windowless rooms furnished with a handful of desks, old schoolhouse chairs, and a typewriter. There were twenty or so men there. Big men. One approached immediately. "Hey, welcome, welcome," he said, as if I were the most important guest at a banquet.

A full half of Greenhaven's population are men sentenced to life in prison. *Life* is a misnomer. The men will actually qualify to participate in the parole process, but first must be incarcerated for at least twenty-five years. While some of the lifers were in for kidnapping or something perverse, most were in for murder. Usually of a spouse, friend, or an unfortunate drug acquaintance. Most of the men going up for parole had been caught at lesser offenses, usually drug dealing or stealing in one form or another. One burly little man told me that he stole only BMWs. He was very proud of that.

A handful of lifers staffed Greenhaven's Prerelease Center. Prerelease was designed to prepare inmates for possible parole. The lifers taught potential parolees how to interview successfully at parole board hearings and how to find jobs and residences. For the lifers, working in the center was an earned honor. Unlike inmates working in the machine shop, the laundry, or the kitchen, the prerelease center staff set their own schedule and goals. To get these jobs the lifers needed spotless in-house records and, preferably, education. Most of the staff had bachelor's or master's degrees from a local university.

I volunteered at Greenhaven for eighteen months during my sophomore and junior years of college. I was supposed to represent the outside world and was charged with giving the men feedback about how they could present themselves most effectively to interviewers, employers, and parole officers. Instead, I spent most of my time telling the inmates how much things cost and what people were doing with their hair.

I tried to appear unafraid around the large men, but it took effort. I couldn't decide who frightened me more, the guards or the inmates. Both were large and had rippled arms and practiced sneers. To combat my fears I befriended a few men. One, Ernest Morton, was a lifer who had kidnapped someone. Everyone called him Spank. When I was skeptical about an inmate's story, I'd ask Spank and he'd tell me which parts to believe.

We didn't have many chances to talk when I was there, so through a series of letters, spanning the eighteen months I worked there, Spank interpreted the prison culture for me. For example, he told me why so many of the men wore watches and checked them so frequently. If I was incarcerated, I speculated, I wouldn't pay any attention to time. Spank disagreed. "You can't do your entire stretch at once. Doing time is a matter of doing a little bit of it at a time. When you feel down, you just get through the day. If that's too much you get through one hour, or the next ten minutes, or the next twenty seconds, and you time it." He also told me about the importance of respect, and about the Aryan Nation and Black Muslims, and about how men could get better-quality drugs inside the prison than outside.

I was especially curious about the men going up for parole. They chain-smoked. They couldn't sit still. They asked the same questions over and over. They picked fights. I wondered why they were nervous. If I were them, I thought, I'd be excited to be so close to getting out. Spank said no. "In here there's someone bringing you food, telling you when to sleep, when to work, when to shit, when to shower, and watching over you. It's addictive. Hard to leave that sometimes."

I didn't understand.

I grew indifferent to the rituals on the transplant unit. Every morning a fleet of doctors appeared at the foot of my bed and inspected me and my chart. Sometimes I slept through it. Other times I asked questions. There were no meals. I was fed through my central line. In the afternoons I scrubbed my mouth and took bedside baths. Terry scrubbed my bald head and arms and legs and belly while I tried not to watch her response to the changes in my body. My once-inquisitive green eyes receded under fleshy cheeks. My limbs grew pale and scrawny. My belly went soft.

To the staff, friends, and family I looked confident. "If anyone can handle this it's you, man," said a friend from graduate school. But late at night there were cracks. After the nightshift settled in I often pulled a pillow over my face and wailed and rocked. Slashing my open hands into the bed. Out of weariness. Out of anger. Out of hunger for the childhood memory of being pulled into my father's chest and protected.

Gradually the days passed. I tried to keep myself occupied when I could think and slept when I could not. My blood counts climbed, signaling the return of my fledgling immune system. I grew strong enough to walk around the room. I nibbled. The nausea and rashes and mouth sores faded.

Then, one morning, the fleet of physicians appeared at the foot of my bed and their leader proudly proclaimed my imminent release. He smiled broadly, his hands hidden in the pockets of his oversized lab coat. I felt like a well-behaved petri dish. I nodded at them, but a disagreeable pang awakened in my belly. He repeated himself as if I hadn't heard him. "You can go home tomorrow!" he said, beaming. Parole.

"Yeah," I said flatly. "Great," I managed to add.

The fleet shuffled out, deflated, denied the celebration they felt they deserved.

———

That night the moon was near full and I couldn't sleep. *What if I get an infection? What if I'm like Jodi and this was all for nothing? What if my body isn't ready? What if I fall and bleed? What if a virus lingering on a doorknob steals its way into my system?*

At three A.M. my exhaustion peaked and I fell into unsettled sleep. At four A.M. Military Mary appeared in my room. Mary, a night nurse, had been in the army. Sometimes she forgot she'd been discharged. I pleaded with her to venture into my space quietly at night, but she'd never change her routine. Without fail, she'd turn on the overheads, assaulting my eyes with bright light. I usually protested aggressively, flailing an arm, "Ahhhh! Mary, what the hell!" but this time I was glad to see her. "Mary?" I whispered. She held my left arm and I heard and felt a blood pressure cuff inflating. Squinting and in need of companionship, I tested the waters. "How's your night going, Mary?" "Fine," she replied. Silence. Pressure on my arm. "One ten over eighty, you're fine. G'night." Her sneakered footsteps retreated and the door closed.

I searched for my central line with my hand, but it was gone. They'd pulled it during the afternoon. My lifeline. I'd only been in the room for thirty days, but it felt as if a year had elapsed. *How long before I feel complete again? When will my hair come back? What will my first shower feel like? What if something happens out there and I can't get back in here fast enough? What if the cancer is still there?*

I was still awake when the first pastel colors of morning lightened the sky. My room slowly brightened and life outside the room grew more boisterous as the morning shift arrived. A large nurse I didn't recognize appeared. She was a little jittery—diet pills, I thought. She produced a sheaf of papers and clicked a pen. "Good morning." All business.

Oh good, I thought, she'll understand what I'm afraid of. She sat down and methodically arranged the papers. She had a routine. She'd done this hundreds of times. *She will help me calm down.*

Her first words were stern and she wiggled a finger in my direction. "It's discharge teaching time. I remind you that you are severely immune-compromised. Because your ability to fight off infection is compromised, you are forbidden from doing, or being near, the following: pets, dust, flowers, fresh fruits, vegetables, shellfish, yogurt, aged cheeses, crowds, children, kissing, sex, swimming in lakes, swimming anywhere there might be—"

"GERMS," I interjected, right on cue.

Germs? Germs? OHMYGOD. There are germs everywhere. In my car, in my shower, in my fridge. No fruits? No swimming? Did she say NO SEX?! When I raised these concerns, she shrugged, annoyed. "You should be excited about leaving." Then she smiled a "Have a nice day" smile like a policeman who's just given you a traffic ticket.

Then it really hit. *They're kicking me out! The insurance companies must have pressured them to dump me and the doctors don't like me anymore and I'm kind of a nuisance . . . but I'm not ready! I know about natural selection. They are leaving me to nature's squadron of viruses and bacteria, who will cull me, one of the weak and infirm, from the herd of my vibrant brethren.* I imagined a fleet of armored germs and bacteria surrounding me, waiting to snatch life away.

"Congratulations." She shook my hand.

A few hours later. Time to go. I puttered around the room as long as I could. There was nothing left but to step outside. I put on a surgical mask to cover my mouth; I would have to wear one whenever I was near people. I gathered around me what courage I could find and—*Oh shit, here we go*—stepped out of the room. The hallway was empty except for a black woman with a wheelchair. She bowed slightly and said, "Your chariot, sir." When I sat, she wheeled me forward toward the elevators. While we waited, she hummed "Amazing Grace."

Amazing Grace, how sweet the sound that saved a wretch like me . . .

The doors opened and she pushed me on. It was just us. A floor below the doors opened and the elevator filled. A little girl, maybe three, stared at me, transfixed. She clung to her mother's leg. I smiled but my mouth was behind the mask.

I once was lost, but now I'm found, was blind but now I see. . . .

At the front door of the hospital Terry met us. The car was running. I stepped outside and a wall of thick humidity pressed into me. I carefully stepped toward the car. The plants in front of the hospital were splashed with a shade of green too bright to be natural. The sky was a fluorescent blue, and even the clouds looked too bright. The wind blew into my face and felt unpredictable after the laminar airflow. My eyes were unaccustomed to adjusting to objects far away and it took longer to focus; the world beyond my immediate surroundings was blurry.

At home, I walked slowly up the stairs to our apartment and in the front door, out of breath. I sat on the couch I'd missed for so long. Fluffed a favorite pillow and then pushed it away. I stood. Eventually I sat down and fidgeted with magazines on the coffee table. *The apartment looks bigger than I remember.* I was nervous about everything I touched. *Maybe there is a speckle of bacteria laying in wait there.*

Terry said she was going to the supermarket, we were missing some essentials. I gazed out our rear sliding glass windows and felt my jaw clench. This was the first time I'd be alone. The world was a huge, looming place with threats in every corner. I knew I had to start living again, but I didn't know how. The rules in my old world had changed. Nothing was safe. Supermarkets, movies, and restaurants were all filled with crowds and children. Anything outdoors had bacteria and viruses. I was a prisoner in my own Cloroxed home.

———

During the next three days I moved from the couch only to eat or go to the bathroom. Occasionally, friends from grad school called. I reached into my memory for some hint about what to say, the appropriate inflection, to avoid exposing that I was no longer the same person who had ventured into the transplant unit. I felt like a double, stepping into someone else's life.

I focused on them, asking as many questions as I could. Which professor had screwed over which student? How's your thesis going? Who was at the party? I hoped my barrage of questions would keep them from exposing that I was different now, but I feared I'd convinced no one; I knew I hadn't convinced myself. My words sounded forced, my questions too chipper. But the conversations trickled along anyway. The gap between my life as I'd planned it and the couch where I sat was wide and growing. I began to brood. I brooded well. I brooded in Olympic form.

I ached for my old way of being. The intensity of grad school, the friends, and even the trivial worries. I wanted to worry about flat tires, overdue bills, and grades. The days moved slowly. And this was the great goal, I thought. I watched the sun move across the sky, and the little lizards outside the sliding glass doors, and reruns of inane cop shows. Terror mingled with a heavy, stifling sadness. Smiling and kissing my bald head, Terry offered her encouragement, but it was no use. I was too frightened of exposing myself to something dangerous and too self-pitying to listen. Life was casting me aside.

On the fourth day, at around three in the afternoon, the sky changed colors, as it always did at that time. I was halfway through a rerun, my mind numb, when I noticed it. I walked to the sliding door and peeked skyward. I could see the clouds forming for the afternoon shower. They were dark gray and heavy, massive saturated sponges. I tentatively slid open the glass door, just a crack, and listened to the cacophony of birds and insects. *I need to be careful.*

Standing next to the door, I watched the rerun for a few more minutes until I noticed the birds and insects had quieted. When I turned off the television there was silence. I opened the door a tiny bit more. *Couldn't hurt.* Soon the edges of the clouds were gone. The entire sky was a water-colored, dusky gray. I pulled open the door a little more, and then more, and then peeked out, up into the dark sky. I couldn't resist. I stepped out onto the deck, which looks out over a small pond, a wildlife refuge that was almost always filled with birds of various species. The birds stood silently. I rubbed my bald head and wondered how dangerous it was to stand exposed in the humid air. I must have been surrounded by millions of molds, spores, and fungi. I knew I shouldn't touch anything. *Maybe I should wear a mask to cover my mouth out here?*

Then a sole raindrop landed on my head. *Thwap.* It surprised me. How irregular, I thought. Then another on my nose. *Thwap.* I tasted it. *Definitely not smart to drink the rainwater. You're gonna die if you keep this crap up.* Then three more drops landed on my head. *Thwap. Thwap. Thwap.* I giggled.

The sky was almost black. I took off my slippers and ran my feet gently across the warm treated wood of the deck. It was comforting. Raindrops increased. *Thwapthwapthwapthwap.* I wriggled out of my shirt, stretching it over my head, and felt drops on my shoulders and back. They were cold. The birds looked like little statues on the pond. I could see drops on the pond making concentric circles. Each drop did the same as it struck me.

Then CRACK!! A flash of silver lightning punctuated the start of the real downpour. WHOOOOOOSH. I blinked instinctively as the onslaught of pellets struck my chest and dribbled down my abdomen. As the rain intensified, I awkwardly pulled down my pajama bottoms and stood naked in the cool air. Water was everywhere, pinging off of my body and the wood deck and the grass and trees and roof and the birds. And as the torrent soaked my bald head, my chest, and my scrotum, I felt a warm current of soothing energy. It started in my wet feet and ascended through my body; a pure bursting, primitive wonder like my first orgasm, it bubbled out of my throat with an open guttural release. My mouth filled with the confluence of salty tears and fresh rain and I raised my arms and squinted skyward and laughed and screamed and cried and drank.

Food Appreciation

I can admit it now. Before the bone marrow transplant I was an anti-vegan of the worst kind. I only ate things that had faces or could run away from me. Of course, I never killed anything myself other than a vegetable, I'd never kill a living thing, but I didn't think twice about eating things other people killed.

Don't get me wrong, I never had many burgers or steaks, but not because of some deep respect for cows or things bovine. It was more because I liked poultry. Birds. Perhaps my parents' bird-watching was genetically expressed in me differently. Instead of wanting to see and understand birds, I wanted to eat them.

And I always ate fast. Food was not a hobby. I didn't mind eating, but I never particularly enjoyed it either. It was a chore, something to get done. Friends teased me that I ate faster than anyone they knew. This became a source of pride.

During the bone marrow transplant I lost most of my taste buds. The only thing left was texture. After a month of not eating, I started reintroducing foods slowly. Soup. Rice. But eating was largely unsatisfying. My brain said *soup*, but my mouth said *water*. My brain said *rice*, and my mouth said *packing material*. So I escalated to spicier foods. Terry cooked jambalaya, a spicy Cajun dish. I asked her why she put peanuts in it. She told me they weren't peanuts, they were peppers. Nothing tasted like it should.

After a week at home, I decided I wanted to go out and see the world again. The first place I wanted to see was the supermarket. I didn't know why. I just wanted to visit the food, like an old friend who's been away. I donned a Red Sox cap to hide my shiny bald head, and put on the mouth mask I was ordered to wear to shield me from germs. Then, in the middle of a workday afternoon, I drove to the Winn Dixie.

The Winn Dixie is huge. Walking in, I was greeted by a cool produce breeze. When I was in high school I worked pushing carts, bagging groceries and cleaning up spills in a local supermarket. When the mayonnaise jar broke I cleaned it up. When too many carts collected in front of the First Colonial Bank and the Caldor's I retrieved them. When Ms. Marsh needed her cart pushed to her car I dutifully walked it out. The smells of supermarkets, from the clean wet air of produce to the dank musty smell of wet cardboard in the back rooms, are familiar, even comforting.

I walked into the Winn Dixie and started in the bakery. Fresh bread. Two women were putting out loaves; one dropped them in white bags while the other put orange price labels on them. They were stacked in front of the display case and I squeezed a few for good measure. Soft. The crust crackled and snapped with the pressure. I continued. Down the way the sweets were displayed. Cannoli, cookies filled with chocolate and berries, and powdered sugar surprises. Each item sat on its own frilly paper carpet as if it were a presentation to the queen.

I cut through the alcohol section, stopping only for a moment to review the mixes. Margarita and whiskey sour mix, piña colada

and White Russians. I passed a reasonable assortment of wines
and beers, including my old favorite Black and Tan. Then to the
dairy aisle. I've never known much about cheeses. I picked up the
small cheese bricks, one at a time, and studied them. The Brie,
pepperjack, cheddar, and spicy dill, each with its own density, its
own color, and its own consistency. The pepperjack had green
and red pepper turning this way and that, the cheddar was light
orange through and through. The soft Brie wore its white skin like
a winter coat. I squeezed a little too hard and the cellophane
wrapping bristled. I put it down.

Margarines, butters, creams, and spreads, each boasting its
own special properties for cooking, flavoring, or topping. Then
down the pasta aisle. Rigatoni. Macaroni. Spaghetti. Farfalle. The
rigatoni had stripes; someone had taken the time to make the
machines cutting the rigatoni carve stripes. Down the aisle I
found the close relatives of good pasta in bottles and jars. Pesto,
tomato sauce and three cheese mixes. I examined the pesto ingredients carefully, making sure they were all there. Olive oil, pine
nuts, basil leaves, shallots. It was a small cardboard box with a see-
through plastic enclosure. It was too soft. Pesto should be a solid, I
thought, not a liquid.

Back up the aisle, the spices with their multicolored tops
caught my eye. Jars just thin enough to fit perfectly in my palm.
Coriander, paprika, oregano, tarragon, nutmeg. I noticed that
spices beginning with C can be hot. Chili pepper. Cayenne
pepper.

I passed the poultry displayed in freezers, the white ice gathering thick on the steel rail. Wings, thighs, breasts, legs. Mixed or
segregated. Skinned, boned, or whole. Labels advertising percent-
ages of fat in each piece. I imagined breaded baked chicken. Near
the meat case there were new grills displayed. One was set up with
plastic food on the grill. The plastic chicken leg was dwarfed by a
plastic hamburger.

I skipped paper products and magazines and toured the jellies and marmalades, jams and preserves. Honey. Strawberry. Blueberry. Boysenberry. Multiberry! Shades of blue and dark red, purple and honey orange. For a moment I contemplated opening the honey right there, listening for the vacuum pop of an open jar and licking the jar rim as Pooh Bear might. Surely the honey would taste like it should! I set the jar down, and before I walked away, I ran my hand along the label as if I were touching a lover.

I spent the most time in the snack food aisle. Pretzels in knots, or strings, or cigar style. Salted or not. Unsalted? What's the point? Popcorn. Smartfood. Chips for dipping. Corn chips, tortilla chips, and Doritos. Potato chips. Ruffled, straightened, or curved in long cans. I picked up a few of the puffy bags and studied the contents. Huge chips on top giving way to smaller and smaller ones deeper into the bag, as if the little ones were hiding. I could almost feel the texture in my mouth. The snap of a chip and the salt that opens a flood of taste across the tongue and cheeks. I've always thought that people can be broken into three categories. There are salt people, sweet people, and carbo people. Sure, some folks dip into more than one category, but if you force them to choose, say they only get one food on a deserted island and don't have to worry about nutrition, they can make the choice. I'm a salt person. I lingered in the aisle, studying colors and shapes.

I ended the trip in the produce section. Squeezed the grapefruit. Too soft. Good self-respecting grapefruit are firm and sport a thin skin. The grapes looked good. Snappy and bright green. As though they might suddenly burst out of their plastic bags and run about the store. There was a special on cherry tomatoes. Fire red. Dense. I rolled one in my palm. The carrots had been picked over, but the oranges and lemons looked healthy. I tossed a lemon from behind my back and almost lost it in the avocados. I put it back.

I left through the electronic out door, headed back into the oppressive humidity. No purchases made. But a new admiration for food. And a determination. I'd never eat a fast meal again. As soon as my taste buds were back, I'd eat all of it. Slow. One bite, one lick, one swallow at a time. Hmmmm.

Blazers

Calico Jack's Oyster Bar was alive with the euphony of Saturday-afternoon revelers. Ceiling fans slowly turned in the smoky heat. The ornate dark wooden banisters running throughout the room glistened with sweat. Trim young waiters and waitresses bounded to and fro, heaving beer mugs and plates of Calico Jack's dangerous wings and other deep-fried atrocities.

Calico Jack's chicken wings were not ordinary. They were rated on five levels. When waiters brought a plate of wings it had a small flag standing in the middle, with the level of hotness displayed in bold letters. The mildest wings were called Fiery. The next three levels, in ascending order, were Searing, Scorching, and Blistering. The final level, rumored to be unfit for human consumption, was Blazing. According to legend, Blazers were basted in a distilled paste of imported peppers so hot they had to be handled with thick gloves, lest one's hands swell up.

My table was packed with friends celebrating my parole from the bone marrow transplant unit. We were in a boisterous mood and I decided it was time to impress the bar. When the waitress asked us for our orders, I asked for Blazers. She stared at me, unimpressed.

"You ever been here before?" she asked, putting a hand on her hip.

When I answered in the affirmative, she droned, "You probably want Scorching wings." The third level. "No one ever orders Blazing wings."

"Blazers!" I insisted, pounding the table like Khrushchev.

She stared. "No, I'm serious, you don't." She had a sorority-girl drawl and practiced attitude.

"Yeah, I do," I demanded.

She growled at me, "Really, it's for your own good, but if you insist, I'll get you some Blisterers, okay?" The fourth level. "They're wildly hot, okay?"

"No, not okay. BLAZERS!"

"Okay, what-e-ver," she answered, shaking her head with pity.

"Blazers or nothing!" I boasted.

"Fine," she answered. "Remember I tried to stop you." As she turned to go, I grabbed her arm.

"Tell the chef I said he's a whining WUSSY."

When the wings came, they had a bright red Blazer flag on them. I'd never seen this particular flag before. The noise in the bar increased as people noticed the flag.

"Hey, those are Blazers!" a guy with a tattoo shouted. He grabbed his girlfriend and a few others and then more people crowded around to see who the fool was. People squeezed in around the table. The plate was dropped in front of me and my friends leaned forward in anticipation. I snatched up the first wing, holding it high in the air. The guy with the tattoo looked transfixed. He slowly shook his head. A girl grimaced. I nibbled and then wolfed it down, then reached for another. The wings were easy to eat. I slurped another and another, each with fanfare. The girl shouted eagerly, the man with the tattoo hollered. A bartender slapped me on the back and brought us a pitcher of free beer.

Of course, only my friends knew that I'd lost all of my taste buds during the bone marrow transplant and couldn't taste the wings. For them, instead of an act of heroism, my eating the wings was only a demonstration of how strongly the transplant had altered me. And as the crowd dispersed I noticed the grins on my friends' faces were gone. They were looking far off. The only sound was the dull hum of a ceiling fan.

Soup

I waited one month and then went back to graduate school part-time. On the first day there was a light rain. I'd just come in to talk to my professors, to arrange to make up the papers and exams I'd missed. The Department of Clinical Psychology is located in the basement of Shands Hospital, where it's impossible to know the weather. When I climbed the stairs to leave I found a large crowd of hospital workers and patients gathered around the double glass doors.

Outside I could see a torrent of rain, water streaming out of the parking lot and into the road. I stood with others staring into the gray scene, unable to see more than one hundred feet through the squall. People near me clutched umbrellas. A short, older man, wearing a green scrub top, held a *Harper's* magazine over his head and laughed before racing into the downpour. Umbrella-less, I stood awhile, waiting for a break before walking home. Eventually the rain turned a little softer and a group of us headed out.

I'd gone a hundred feet or so when I saw a yellow-raincoated figure, maybe three feet tall, hopping in and out of puddles on the sidewalk. An adult with an umbrella stood nearby. I couldn't see the face, the gender or any other characteristics of the little person, but I guessed he or she was four or five years old. I could see muddy yellow boots and a raincoat with buckles and big pockets. Small hands emerged from the sleeves. The little being gathered together all of its energy, sprung into the air, hovered—defying gravity—and then crashed into the puddles, sending water everywhere. An infectious, high-pitched giggle erupted. The little hands waved faster, excited.

And for the first time ever, I felt an unexpected impulse. The desire to jump in the puddles, too. Gather the child in my arms, bring him home, towel him off, and feed him some soup.

Dictated Chart Note

The patient had an autologous bone marrow harvest. Due to the low number of mononuclear cells present following the first harvest he required a second bone marrow harvest. The patient was then admitted for autologous bone marrow transplant and received high dose Cytoxan and VP-16 chemotherapy.

Patient then underwent a reinfusion of both autologous bone marrow harvests. The patient encountered common post-transplant complications including mylosuppression requiring blood transfusions, rashes secondary to antibiotics, fevers with neutropenia, nausea, vomiting, and diarrhea. This represented a fairly uncomplicated post-transplant course. He was discharged from the bone marrow transplant unit after an approximate 4 week hospitalization. He will remain in limited isolation at home and be seen frequently in the outpatient bone marrow transplant clinic. It is believed that following this transplant the patient has a significant chance at cure (five year disease-free survival) of at least 40%.

CHARLES ERIC SCHULMAN, M.D.
Shands Hospital at the University of Florida

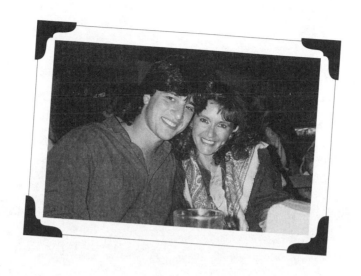

Part Four

Respite

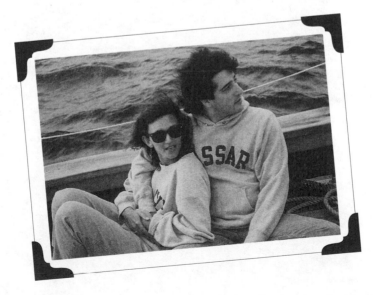

Ron

As the sun descends, the winter sky is streaked with gentle pastels. Pinks, oranges, blues. The trees have shed the snow from yesterday, but the ground wears a white-powdered blanket. With the wind it feels Arctic cold and the temperature is working to stay above zero. Since the transplant I've been more sensitive to cold. I suspect this has something to do with my lack of hair.

It will take us forty minutes to get from the airport in Indianapolis to Bloomington, where Terry grew up. Ron, Terry's father, is driving. We are rumbling along, heat on full blast, in a pickup truck. I've been staring at the erratic ice circles clinging just beyond the reach of the wipers. I'm not looking forward to unpacking our luggage. It's covered by a plastic tarp in the bed of the truck. It's going to be very cold.

When I first met Ron one year ago, my hair was graduate-student long, down near my shoulders. We were at a stoplight coming back from the airport, minutes after we'd met, when he reached over to me and put a finger in my long hair, curling it around. "I dunno, Dan, your hair is awful long," he'd said quietly. But now, five months after the transplant, my hair is military short, and he hasn't said a word about it, my prognosis, or anything else about my illness.

To Ron, I'm a city boy. In the past he's enjoyed teasing me about my lack of knowledge about horse feed, corn growth cycles, and my inability to put a spark plug within a mile of its proper home in a tractor. And I've given him a hard time about his inability to beat me at Indiana bocce, a game I adapted from the old Italian men's version. In Indiana bocce competitors use an acre of backyard and attempt to throw old croquet balls closest to a marker, usually a softball. "You can just write me a check this year, Ron," I used to tease.

But as we rumble along, Ron stares straight ahead. I feel a tingle in my shoulders. A tightness. I'm nervous. I don't want him to treat me differently, but he already has. There's been no city-boy teasing. No comments about my shoes, lousy sense of direction, or lack of hair. I peek at him as he drives. He's unblinking, his gloved right hand wrapped on the wheel, his left in his lap. His face seems frozen except for the pools of pink heat in the skin beneath his jaw. I suddenly want to yell out, "Stop the truck! I'm gonna run home!" Show him how strong I am. But I look back at the wipers, watch the rhythm, and lean my head against the side window, which is a mistake because it's cold.

During my last three visits he's invited me into the pickup truck to go somewhere. I no longer ask him where we're going, I know better. He won't answer. Once we found a dirt road and followed it ten miles to a small cemetery filled with the names of my wife's relatives, the babies who died in childbirth, the men who died before the women. Another time we found the limestone quarry and drove around the long fence of slabs surrounding the plant. Like an enormous Indiana Stonehenge, massive stones reach into sky.

I enjoy our trips. The hum of the engine, the feel of Ron's lined canvas jackets he always loans me. I like the comfortable silence. The eventual teasing. But this year he knows I'm more fragile. He lunged forward and scooped the bags from me at the airport. The needle scars on my hand are obvious. My puffy face. I caught his glances. He's noticed my shivering, my weakness.

Days pass. Ron is still silent. There's no conversation at dinner. No competitive banter in the living room. I try to engage him. We're washing dishes when I put a damp hand on his shoulder.

"I noticed you've been avoiding talking to me about bocce this time, Ron. You know, I am a psychologist in training, I might be able to help you work through your fear of me—" but I start coughing after the last word and he tries to smile, but at first his lips won't join him. "You could just write me a check, Ron," I say when my voice returns. He asks if I'm okay. I nod. I go back to drying the dishes.

"I hope you're better at psychology than you are bocce," he mutters, smiling.

I'm in the living room the next day, surfing channels, when I overhear Barb, Terry's mom, "Don't you do anything that makes him sick, Ronny," and a moment later he bounds into the living room.

"Meet me at the truck." And a heavy canvas jacket lands in my lap.

I hear Barb's voice from the kitchen: "Dan, you don't have to go with him."

I scamper out into the waiting pickup truck, careful not to slip on the ice in my loafers. I slide into the seat and immediately notice the cold through my jeans. My ankles are freezing. The snow is back, though just a dusting; most of the sky is clear. Occasional puffy flakes swirl in midair, in no particular rush to reach the ground. We drive for a while and then Ron abruptly pulls into a long driveway. A dairy farm? I've never been to one before. It has all of the classic farm accoutrements—a huge red barn, a little white house, long mazes of fencing and feeding troughs disappearing into the distance. Cows litter the scene; most lounge lazily in the snow. There are industrial-looking buildings nearby.

The truck negotiates a series of ruts and snowy mounds and settles, stalling asleep, next to a row of other pickup trucks.

The smell is distinct and immediate. Cows. Cow food, cow sweat, cow dung. I follow Ron closely over bulldozed humps of snow and around a tractor whose innards lie in a neat row, beneath snowy hats. I am silently lamenting my choice of footwear as Ron pulls open a door and yells, "Hey, Cujo!" and steps inside a porch. As I follow him into the darkness, a mangy creature leaps, growling, toward my chest. A wolf? I cover my throat reflexively.

"Gee, Dan, he's just saying hello, he won't kill ya." When my eyes adjust I can see Ron holding a beagle by the collar, petting him aggressively. "He's just a cute little fella, aren't ya, Cujo?" My heart pounds in my chest. I pull the wool hat down over my ears.

Post-Cujo we walk down the narrow corridor toward a great rumbling sound. We emerge into a small square concrete room. In the center of the room there's a pit where two men stand, moving quickly. Above them, on long cement ramps, cows stand in gated cubicles. The men in the pit are connecting udders to long hoses that gyrate. The sound is terrific. Cows are singing, machines are chugging, and Cujo is howling behind us somewhere. Ron yells to the men, "How's it goin', Shorty? Gerry?"

Shorty and Gerry are wearing heavy rubber overalls and calf-length boots. They're covered with cow fluids of one sort or another. Ron puts his arm around me and leans close to my ear to point out how the machines work. Then gates open and new cows move into place. The men quickly attach hoses.

Ron waves at the men and smiles and they respond in kind. He leans into me again, and his hand lands on my wool hat. He rubs my head affectionately.

"That's where milk and ice cream come from, Dan," he says, chuckling. "Now I've got a special surprise. Come on," he yells. I scamper behind him and am just close enough to hear him yell over his shoulder, "I want to show you where we get fertilizer. . . ."

Laboratory Coats

As it turns out, carrots are not brain food. At least not for me. I discovered this while sitting in the cafeteria at Shands Hospital. I was back, enrolled full time, in graduate school. Following my stint in the bone marrow transplant unit, I got started on my dissertation.

I'd noticed that my mood had an effect on how sick I became during chemotherapy and thought this might be an interesting thing to research for my dissertation. The American Psychological Association agreed and offered modest financial support. On this particular day I was in the cafeteria, huddled over notebooks and journal articles. The large room buzzed like a summer playground, with laughter and chatter and urgency. I work well in places where sound ebbs and flows; I guess I find the sound soothing. Perhaps more important, in cafeterias I'm allowed to snack while I work, unlike in libraries, where book police seize hapless pretzels at the first crunch.

An older student, Sandy, had advised me to choose a dissertation idea I loved. "Without love, or a real hunger to know the outcome, leaping through the academic hoops necessary to complete a dissertation resembles wading through a mosquito-infested swamp," he'd advised. "You'll do anything to escape." But on this morning, despite my love for the project, my mind wandered. I'd read twenty journal articles and they were all starting to fade together despite my careful note-taking. I was in a corner of the cafeteria near the tray-return conveyor belt and could see the entire room. It was eleven o'clock or so, still too early for the lunch rush but starting to fill up. There were a number of elderly couples, a few young mothers with babies and crying toddlers, and a smattering of young physicians. Two of them near me, clean-shaven men, caught my eye. They wore long laboratory coats and were standing in front of the tray return.

The length of a laboratory coat in many teaching hospitals signifies position in the academic hierarchy. Medical students wear coats that are almost vests, trim affairs that barely run south of their waists. It makes them look as if they should be serving wine. Interns, also called first-year residents, have coats that are slightly longer, just below the butt, and residents' coats go to the thigh. The coat of an attending physician, the highest rung on the ward ladder, may drop as low as the calf. Particularly short attendings sometimes have coats that drag on the floor. Once, while wandering the fifth floor of Shands Hospital, I swore I saw an attending stride down the hall with two little boys carrying the hem of his coat behind him.

These two attendings were young, perhaps thirty-five, and had coats that were too long for their bodies. The thinner one wore two beepers. He had a bald spot, but he'd shaved his remaining hair very short. He had tiny horn-rim glasses and stroked his chin with one hand, just his thumb and pointer, while his other hand shook in midair, fingers all outstretched. He was making a point. The other man was even shorter and carried his weight in his belly. His fingers were tucked inside his lab-coat pockets, but his thumbs drummed his belly. He was nodding, serious.

They were discussing a medical point. I could almost feel the thin one presenting evidence. He'd figured something out about a patient, something important that someone else had missed. He was delineating each symptom, each clue for his colleague, who was enjoying the careful presentation. While I nibbled a carrot I watched, admiring. There was something awe-inspiring about two men dedicating even their free time to their patients. I've always been impressed with passionate people, those who throw themselves into their work with abandon. These two were such physicians.

Then I saw a third man approaching them. He walked slowly, too slowly, carrying his empty lunch tray far out in front of him. He was large and his gray-speckled hair went this way and that. I could see half of his face from where I sat. It was puffy, covered with stubble and pockmarks. He was not wearing a laboratory coat. He had on dark gray pants that weren't hemmed, institutional issue. And a thin white button-down shirt with collars too wide for the current fashion. What was he doing? Why would he walk right toward these two scholars with so little regard for their important conversation?

Then I saw his cane. Long and white with the red stripe. He held it in his right hand. As he approached the two physicians with his lunch tray, hoping to return it, the two parted, each stepping back a few feet, leaving him the steel rail. My stomach dropped. The doctors stopped talking, regarding the blind man with a casual indifference, as if they were watching a stage play. The blind man knew they were there, he'd heard them as he approached. He stopped. Where do I return my tray? he seemed to be asking. He took a step forward, and another. Then another. The two doctors didn't move toward him or speak. They watched. By now my heart was pounding. I stood up and started toward them, but it was too late. The blind man took another step, larger, and pounded into the tray-return rail with the clank of plastic against metal. He dropped like a car over a precipice, limbs rising in surprise. For a moment there was nothing, a quiet silence, and I noticed cafeteria food littering his legs and face and the rail.

Suddenly there was commotion. A familiar black face from the cafeteria staff—I'd seen him serve potatoes with strong hands and a friendly nod—appeared and called out the blind man's name. He rushed forward, between patients and around a wheelchair, gracefully gathering the tray from the floor and easily lifting the big man to his feet.

The two doctors came back together like a curtain dropping. They stood in front of the blind man and resumed their conversation. Fingers snapped back inside of laboratory coats. Thumbs drummed away. A hand shook in midair while another stroked a pointed chin.

Animal

Atavan, Demerol, Percocet, and morphine. In the course of treatment I had them all and each one was a slightly different voyage. I'd ride the warmth in my chest, akin to drinking rum, and enjoy the soft release of all things material and inconsequential. Suddenly there were no scratches on life's veneer. No ego handcuffs, no weeds. All was as smooth and still as winter ice.

After one of my biopsies, Laura, my favorite anesthesiologist, left me with a patient-controlled morphine pump. I could administer as much or as little as I wanted within broad limits. We both knew I wouldn't abuse it. When I pushed the button, the little machine had the friendliest sound, a light chime like a small Chinese gong.

As the pain subsided over the next few days, I pushed the button less and less. But each time the gong chimed I enjoyed the tide of warmth and comfort that flooded through me with the opiate.

Eighteen months later I was standing in front of an elevator in Shands Hospital. I pushed the up button. When the car arrived it chimed, that same wonderful sound. . . . Suddenly the familiar warmth flooded my chest and expanded, eager, through every extremity. I stepped on the elevator carefully, leaned against the wall, feeling dreamy and content, my knees weak and swirling.

I like to pretend that I'm not a member of the animal kingdom. That a chemical couldn't totally alter my emotional responses. That I couldn't be conditioned to life's stimuli like a pigeon or dog, psychology's favorite animals. I'm above conditioned responses. *I've got free will, after all! I make choices!*
      But I suspect that whenever I hear that chime . . .
      Ahhhh.

Jacob's Exit

It took a while, but eventually I was ready to see patients again. It was challenging. Years later I would learn to tell patients that I, too, had been through a cancer experience, but months after the transplant, when I was just venturing back into those rooms as a young professional, I was still too raw. When patients asked if I understood their experience I felt the hot flash of an airport searchlight, it blinded me. I knew that if I told them of my transplant I'd be unable to concentrate, too lost in my own worries. I started slowly and was soon seeing many of the patients admitted to the bone marrow transplant unit.
      I'd found a niche. The patients seemed to benefit from talking with me. One of them was Jacob. He was a few years younger than me and also had Hodgkin's disease. From his medical chart it was apparent that he had an aggressive form of the

disease. Before the transplant his lymphatic system was rife with tumors.

Jacob was a sports fan. His room was covered with posters of football heroes and basketball stars. He had a short-wave radio in his room and spent hours listening to sporting events in Miami, Jacksonville, and Orlando. Sometimes when I came into his room he would shush me with a cough so he could hear a play or a commentator's energetic words.

For one month I visited every few days. We talked about college football, how his mother was doing, how he could have a little more patience with the nurses, and when he might get out. Jacob talked with his entire body. I remember him teaching me about college football — "Listen up now, Emmitt Smith or no, this year Georgia's going to pulverize Florida," and his arms waved through the air as if he were conducting an aria. When he laughed he opened an ugly mouth wide and I could see his extensive bridgework. A hairy belly bounced.

Over time his cough worsened. He had a fungal infection in his chest and amphotericin B, a tough drug, had little impact. I sat across from him one afternoon thinking that he was going to die, that this big guy in front of me, so full of electric animation, was running out of time. I was thankful that he could not read my thoughts.

They told Jacob that things didn't look good and that his blood counts weren't returning. That the fungal infection he was fighting could be unrelenting. I was officially off the hook because as a psychologist, my role was not to give him medical information, but to help him cope with whatever challenges he faced. But he studied me anyway and gauged the truth by watching my gestures, my playfulness, my good-byes. One afternoon, when his cough made it almost impossible for him to communicate, he said, "I'm down in the fourth quarter, huh?" He studied me as I told him I didn't know.

———

A few mornings later I came to see Jacob. I washed my hands as always. I stepped into the room. His bed was gone. The room was empty. Immaculate. Silent. No posters of Larry Bird or Magic Johnson on the walls. No Joe Montana. And no Jacob. The room had been cleaned thoroughly and quickly of any hint of him. Even the electric cords running from the laminar airflow had been scrubbed and shined black. Then my legs felt heavy and I sat down, cross-legged, on the floor. I wanted to write something on the walls. Some message about Jacob. Who he was. Or how he'd spent time here. The way he held that radio in his lap or waved his arms. And maybe a message about me. About the gnawing relief and guilt in my stomach for surviving when he hadn't, like a terrible hunger. But I didn't. I had another patient to see.

Mixed Blessings

I like what it did to me.

I like that I remember how my heart pounded in my ears when I forced my feet to step on the winter New England ground, a wool cap covering my bald scalp. That memory helps now, helps me discern fear of real danger from fear of tragedies I've invented.

I like that I remember kneeling on the linoleum like a wrestler in starting position, in front of the toilet, understanding the rhythm of chemotherapy's assault on my rib cage. It helps me celebrate my body now, when I do a deep limbering stretch or when I run.

I like that I remember the vulnerability in my thighs and knees when I stumbled out after being diagnosed. How it keeps life's smaller disappointments from growing.

I like that I remember how badly I longed for trivial worries. How I wanted to obsess about a flat tire, or a maligning, throat-tightening remark from a colleague, or a bill long overdue. It lets me play in trivialities without getting lost in them.

I only wish the memories could be evacuated from my dreams. I'm tired of the haunting explosions into wakefulness, bolt upright at three A.M., raising my arms to protect myself from unseen demons.

A Roller Coaster

Terry loves roller coasters. I discovered this trait early in our relationship when she convinced me to ride every coaster at the Paramount King's Island Park in Ohio, where one of her sisters lives. The park had six roller coasters, including a steel one that turned and twisted over a forest, a wooden one modeled after the old Coney Island coasters that shook and rattled, and one that looped a few times to shake out any spare change. I went on all of them with her, afraid of losing masculinity points if I stood and waved from a bench near the ride. Since then we've ridden coasters from coast to coast and in a few other countries. The coaster inside the mall in Edmonton, Canada, was the hardest. After getting off the coaster I realized the Canadians must have looser regulations than we do regarding top speeds allowed on their coasters. We sat in the front, the only riders. It hit mach 1. My cheeks blew open and my eyes filled with a protective coat of water. After the ride, when the steel seat belt opened, releasing us, I got out and checked behind me, suspecting I might have left something in the seat. Like, perhaps, my liver. Terry, sniffling, her eyes still tearing, said, "Let's do it again," and I told her she could just strap me to the front bumper of the car on the way back to the hotel.

Of course I wouldn't ride if I didn't enjoy them. The rush of speed, the rattling of the cars as they shake or sway. The fear that this will be the time that the car breaks from the track and sails into the afternoon sky. It's a fun fear, a playful fear. A worry instantly and completely evaporated by the slow braking of the cars as they settle into the last gentle slope before stopping. When everyone on the coaster looks at the person sitting with them and smiles.

So naturally, when we visited Busch Gardens, a Tampa-area theme park, we had to ride the coasters. A few times. Busch Gardens is unique in the Florida theme-park world. Unlike Disney and Epcot, or the movie production company parks, Busch Gardens is a theme park that caters to families but whose parent company actually focuses on beer, the central product of the Anheuser-Busch bottling company. It's created some complicated marketing problems for them. As part of the experience we toured the factory that makes the beer and listened as the tour guide explained how the barley and hops and yeast work together to produce the "greatest beverage ever concocted." I watched the steel rails and bottles sliding along, getting labeled and filled with beer, and wondered how a mouse could have ever gotten into one of the bottles, one of my favorite urban legends.

Then we got to sample the beer, Busch beer and Budweiser and Michelob and even some of the Natural Light, a new especially watery beer they'd just introduced. They gave us the beer in small paper cups that reminded me of pee cups at the internal medicine clinic. We had a few and then decided to hit some of the rides. The lines went fast. I finished my last cup just as we got onto the Python, which advertised a seventy-foot drop. I was a little nervous. Terry smiled at me as we were strapped in and our car started its slow ascent. Just as the coaster neared the first peak, and I could see each letter on the sign at the top that said, PLEASE KEEP HANDS INSIDE THE COASTER AT ALL TIMES, I felt a sharp gnawing in my shoulder. I realized immediately what the pain meant. I watched Terry as we reached the apex. She smiled at me and then looked straight ahead, throwing her arms into the air. As the car shot down I watched her curly hair lift and bounce, black with streaks of red, along her cheeks and neck.

I felt my heart slowing. I wanted to worry about the speed or the turns, the drops or abrupt swings. I tried to force myself to focus on the rickety wooden planks holding up the rails of the coaster, but I couldn't muster even a sparkle of nervousness. My body relaxed. Terry's fists were clenched, her face tight, her eyes wide. As the ride progressed I rubbed my shoulder and looked into the sky. There were low cumulus clouds. I wondered if it would rain soon. *The pain in my shoulder is not in my head. This is really happening.* It wasn't a muscle ache, or a strain, it was the familiar deep bone gnawing, caused by only one thing. And then I remembered the nightmares I'd been having. It all clicked.

Eventually the coaster slowed. Stopped. Terry looked at me curiously. I pasted on a smile and lied, "Come on, wasn't that great? Let's do it again."

Jennings

"What might this be?" I asked, and handed the piece of cardboard, covered with a printed inkblot, to the patient. I was just starting my second year of graduate school, before the bone marrow transplant, when I was still healthy. The patient studied it for a few moments and then answered, his voice wavering, "That's an angry, beautiful ape, wearing a bathrobe." I wrote down his response and asked him what else he saw. "He's holding a staff in his hand, striking himself." I showed him the next card. And the next.

When the patient and I were finished I sequestered myself in the student room and scored all of the testing materials, organized my notes, and went over everything a second time just to be sure. Then I began to compile the information I had. The patient's testing showed an average I.Q., but his vocabulary scores were considerably higher than scores on tests requiring sustained concentration. A number of things could cause this. I guessed that psychopathology or a learning problem might be suppressing his intellectual functioning and that his actual I.Q. might be higher. His scores on the MMPI, a widely used true-false test, confirmed this suspicion. This test suggested that the patient was severely depressed and had some psychotic thinking. I considered what I'd learned from my ninety-minute interview with him. For the first time in the patient's life he'd realized he was attracted to men. He was a devout Christian, married and a respected member of his church, and his fierce desire to be sexual with men had spun him into a dark depression. Then I looked over his scores and responses to the Rorschach. I didn't know what to do with them. My research mentor, a behaviorist, had told me he thought the Rorschach inkblot test was "bullshit." No test in psychology had been studied as frequently or with as much acrimony. But I was doing this assessment under the supervision of Dr. Jennings, a dynamic supervisor and the oldest member of the faculty. It was my first assessment for him and I wanted to impress him. Older students told me the Rorschach was his favorite test.

The scoring system for the Rorschach in vogue at the time was the Exner system. It required a complicated set of calculations and decisions about each response along a number of dimensions. When I tallied everything the scoring suggested that the patient might be suicidal. I didn't know what to make of the actual content of the patient's responses and was nervous about drawing too many conclusions given what my research mentor had told me. I put it all together and jotted down a note on a card to prompt me when I was with Dr. Jennings. "Patient bisexual or gay, suicidal, probably above average intelligence."

I found Dr. Jennings's office, took a deep breath, and knocked. A gruff "Yes?" answered and I entered. I sat down and Dr. Jennings looked at me. I started to describe the session, "I saw the patient on the eighth floor and as expected he appeared despondent and demonstrated a slowing of—" Dr. Jennings's gruff voice interrupted, "Whoa, whoa, whoa. Slow down, Shapiro. Just read me card four." And he waved both his hands at me as if I'd sneezed on him.

"Dr. Jennings?" I asked.

"Verbatim, Shapiro. Read me what the patient said verbatim, you know, without commentary. I want to know exactly what the patient said to card four on the Rorschach. The father card."

I set the folder on my lap and searched my papers. I found the verbatim responses to each card and read what the patient had said, about the ape in the bathrobe. Jennings squinted. Looked from me to the ceiling. Then back at me.

"Ooooh. That's bad. He's bisexual and confused, not happy about it. Anguished. A religious guy. He try to kill himself?"

I swallowed hard. When I was eleven or so, I used to go into New York City with my father and a friend. We'd go to the magic stores and watch young magicians who worked there, sometimes buy a trick or two. I loved the blue velvet they put on the countertops, the polished coins that disappeared, the bright silks that appeared in my pocket and in a book across the room. Sitting in front of Jennings, I felt that same sense of wonder. "Do it again," I wanted to say. And time after time he did. He told me when my patients were suicidal, when they were about to drop out of therapy, or when they had a crush on me. He traced patient hints like a man who finds water with a divining rod.

During that second year of school, rumors started that Dr. Jennings was going to step down as director of the clinical program. He disappeared first for a few weeks, and then again for a few months. Eventually an older student told me about his ill health, a tumor, and a recovery. And then he was back, and I lined up to get therapy supervision from him, not knowing when he might suddenly decide to retire.

I'd never felt as naked.

Sitting in the little white room with Jennings I was a microbe under a massive magnifying lens. It didn't help that he put nothing on his walls or his desk.

"Patients are free to project themselves into the space this way," he explained.

There were no distractions in the office. No trinkets, no landscape prints, no family photographs. And the same for conversation. In the pool of human interchange, with Jennings there was no shallow end. No way to warm up one's toes first, ease in up to the calves, and then dunk under. It was dive in or nothing. And sitting on the stiff white couch—which reminded me of Nana's house when I was little and "Don't touch anything" rang constantly in my ears—I knew that I would reveal myself no matter what I said or did. Jennings would turn his gaze in my direction and read me as easily as a billboard along Route 75.

Once a week I sat in his office and discussed one of my patients. For every hour I saw the patient, Dr. Jennings sat with me for a corresponding hour.

My early career in his office was categorized by awkwardness. A typical supervision:

"I'm sorry, it was rude of me," I said.

"What, do you suppose, led you to do it?" Dr. Jennings asked.

"I don't know." I squirmed on the white couch. I'd forgotten about our supervision the previous week. I'd left Dr. Jennings sitting in his office alone without realizing I'd forgotten. I'd even thought about supervision that morning, told Terry not to expect me until six because I'd be with him the last hour of the day, but then I'd left early, not even realizing I was skipping out on supervision with him. And he's the director of the clinical program, I reminded myself. I'd never done it before. I rubbed my head. I couldn't say I'd just forgotten, since in Dr. Jennings's world there was no such thing. We do things for reasons. I watched him as he watched me. He didn't seem angry.

"Honestly, Dr. Jennings, I'm not sure what was going on in my head."

"Well, Shapiro, is that just a wind tunnel sitting on your shoulders today? Do some work. Figure it out." He looked bored.

The patient we were supposed to discuss the week before had blown me off too. I was angry at the patient. I'd sat in the clinic with my door opened while my colleagues took patients into their rooms. There were no messages from him, no notes in my mailbox. The patient was a graduate student in a different department. The odd part was that the week before we'd had an amazing session. The patient had connected his ambivalence about his major professor to his feelings about his own alcoholic father. After the session I'd rushed into the student room and scrawled a point-by-point description of everything said. I'd arrived for supervision five minutes early. When Dr. Jennings's door opened, releasing two haggard supervisees, I was there, clutching my notebook. I stood in his doorway while he reclined, hands behind his balding head, and looked me over.

"Eager to see me today, eh, Shapiro? You're proud of yourself about something. Don't just stand there, come in, come in, I would be cruel to make you wait, wouldn't I?"

I sat down and launched into a description of the session.

But the next week, when I could have used the time even more, to figure out what why the patient didn't return, I'd "forgotten" to see him. It was Jennings's right to be angry, but he wasn't. It was strange. *Why did I avoid Dr. Jennings last week? Think.*

There was silence. He watched me, his hands crossed on his chest. I stared at the thin sprouts of carpet under his chair. They looked like hairs.

The silence gathered mass. I'm never going to be good at this, I thought. *Okay, why would I want to avoid Jennings?*

"Dr. Jennings," I said. "I want to ask a question. How come you don't seem pissed at me for blowing you off last week?"

"You mean the way you're pissed at your patient?" he asked in response.

"Yeah," I admitted. "But you're not at me?"

"Disappointed, but not angry. See, Shapiro, you're just acting your stuff out. I'd be crazy if I took that personally. I don't have control over what you act out. My job is just to help you figure out what *you* were acting out, and what it can teach you."

"Like my job with my patient," I muttered.

"Right. You get pissed. You're wasting your time. Not that patients don't piss us off sometimes, but usually they're just acting out their stuff. Your job isn't to get angry, it's to use whatever they provide to illustrate what they need to learn. Stop being so narcissistic, it isn't all about you. It's about them. Now work, Shapiro. Why'd you miss our supervision? What were you acting out?"

We sat in silence again. Then I spoke.

"I felt rejected," I admitted.

"Shapiro the loser," he said.

"And I was pissed because I'd been working so hard."

"Who does this patient think he is, anyway?"

"And I didn't want to come in here and have you point out to me that I screwed something up," I said.

"It didn't occur to you that last week's session was so intense that the patient must now feel pretty vulnerable to you. That you have too much power and so he tried to teach you that you aren't so important, he doesn't need you, and you took the bait like a catfish."

I sat quietly. *Of course, why didn't I think of that?*

"It's about his vulnerability, Catfish. Not your being a screwup."

I nodded my head. But I also realized I wouldn't have come to it on my own, even if given all of geological time.

"And the bigger picture. You see what I just did with you? To help you figure out why you skipped out on me last week? I haven't taken it personally. This way you have the room to listen to me. I'm not attacking you for your pathology, I'm helping you realize what you did in a way that won't make you defensive. Get it?"

I agreed. But I wasn't sure I got it. Over time it came up over and over. Anything patients did could change my emotional direction. I felt like a little boat with too big a sail. Again and again Jennings pointed out that patients would do with me the same things they did in the world. I needed to stay focused on helping them figure it out and not take it personally.

"Get it?" he'd ask me, after I'd blown off course again. And again. And again.

When I got back from the trip with Terry and the roller coaster, I went in to see my physician. A biopsy followed.

Word of my second relapse arrived on a hot, windy Friday afternoon during my third year of graduate school. I came down to the department from my physician's office eager to share my bad news with someone. I was numb and looking for friends. I told Jennings's secretary and a handful of other people who were still in the department. There were comforting words all around and then Terry and I headed back to our apartment. We'd been there a few hours when the phone rang. It was Jennings. He'd never phoned me before at home.

"Shapiro," he started. "You have to resign from the clinical program. Pursuing more treatment is not consistent with completing your education. Understand? Best of luck," he said. We hung up. I was shocked. It didn't occur to me to argue: that I was ahead of my classmates in completing my thesis; that I had just won research awards from the American Psychological Association; that I had strong clinical and research reviews every year; that NIH was supporting me. I didn't react.

Over the next days our phone rang off the hook. Fellow students first, and then faculty. There were comforting words about my relapse and then angry proclamations about Jennings and the injustice of my termination. A student thought of a protest. A faculty member suggested I should call a lawyer.

"Jennings was a shit who had no right," she'd said. But I didn't feel rage. I felt a strange calm. It wasn't personal. His action wasn't about me.

Dr. Jennings had never shown any sign of disliking me. In fact, he seemed to enjoy bantering with me. And he didn't have enough information about my situation to dismiss me so casually. Something else had to be happening. *Don't react. Think. What's being acted out? What in his life is he expressing? Stay calm. This isn't about me.* It was particularly hard because his dismissal seemed to imply that I wasn't going to live through this relapse. But he didn't know enough about Hodgkin's disease to make that judgment. *See, it isn't about me.*

Eventually it was obvious. This was about Jennings's own illness. *To him,* I thought, *I am the embodiment of vulnerability to illness. A walking reminder that illness can return to anyone at any time. That none of us are immune. And if death can take even the young . . . ,* he must be thinking.

Within a week I was reinstated. Steve Boggs, my major professor, called me and told me my butt still belonged to him. My brief respite from completing my dissertation was over and my position was not in jeopardy. He wouldn't tell me the details, only that he and a few other professors had cornered Jennings and forced the issue. I was relieved to be reinstated. We needed my modest salary. But there was also a stronger pride at something else.

I'm starting to get it.

Satchel's Boomerang

I had a choice. Like Jodi before me, I'd failed a bone marrow transplant. I knew the implications. A logical option was to take credit cards less seriously, drop out of graduate school, and see Tel Aviv and Bangladesh, the Pyramids and Kauai. I could guzzle margaritas and get tattooed, throw wild parties and swim naked. Maybe even get arrested for a noble cause.

The other option was to find the best doctor in the world and try to see him or her. Even thinking about it made me tired. Tired of I.V. poles and polite nurses, insurance letters and scanners. But even more, tired of the world falling away beneath me when near-lethal disappointments struck. Why not turn away from the sterile world of medicine and hardship and live as long as I could? The tumors weren't coming on that quickly, I'd have time. I still felt good.

Satchel Paige, the great black baseball pitcher, used to say about his pitching arm when he wasn't throwing well, "She always comes back, I know she'll be back." My hope was similar. It didn't matter what happened. It always came back. Like a boomerang, the harder I pressed my weight into the throw, the more I thought about traveling and forgetting tumors, the faster hope swooped back.

Saul

Doctors are a strange breed. They nibble at an overwhelming amount of information in medical school. They are too bright to miss the incredible distance between what they know and what there is to know. They dedicate their waking hours to memorizing droplets from a great ocean of information. They learn trivial anatomical structures and then promptly forget them. They stand with groups of more experienced physicians and are asked questions they don't know the answers to. They shake the sleep from their eyes and walk down neon-lit halls feeling inadequate and small. The Ben Casey vision of medicine that propelled them through organic chemistry classes in college crumbles in the face of a reality which includes cureless diseases, obnoxious scut work, and constant humiliation. They wear down. Their lovers wear down and leave them at higher rates than in most professions. The one untarnishable thing they have left is their basic fascination with the human body and what can go wrong inside its miraculous design.

Inevitably, they lose their empathy for pain. The waterfall of pain they hear from countless patients wears them down to smooth rock. After all, they have had to deny themselves so much to succeed. They have endured their own painful humiliation. They have learned that pain is simply a warning mechanism, it isn't real. Is it any wonder that our painful cries empty into a vacuum when doctors are in the room? Is it any wonder that they sometimes forget that we are not our diseases, that to treat our diseases they must also treat us? Is it any wonder that they forget to treat our terror, that they forget to treat our lover's terrors, that they forget that we need soothing and a pat on the shoulder?

Oncologists are drawn to the good fight, to the opportunity to fight a monster on the front line. They are drawn to the magic of rescuing a life from the jaws of the enemy, but soon they find the faces of their patients haunting them. No one has taught them that they need to talk about their losses, that they must mourn the deaths of the patients they grew so fond of. They haven't learned that to survive they must find ways of debriefing themselves. When reaching for the peas at a family dinner, while casually looking into the rearview mirror at a stoplight, or while watching their toddler bound across the kitchen floor, intrusive snapshots of interactions with patients, now dead, sneak into their consciousness. These visions are potent warnings that they should not get too close to their new patients, that they should erect a screen.

But we patients sense these screens. We study these strange beings almost as carefully as we did our first love. Every subtle move of a hand, every nervous cough, every wrinkled brow, captivates us and we play them over and over again in obsessive ruminative detail. Oncologists are our oracles. We wonder if they have seen our futures. We try to engage them, hoping that perhaps an extra few words will help them commit more energy to our struggle.

I always feel a pang when I meet a new oncology fellow. They are new to the front. They have seen the falling shells as residents, but now it will be different. They will have more autonomy. They will make life-altering decisions. They will begin to root for the patients, as much for their own sense of competence as for the patient's health. And when a patient dies, a piece of them will die. They'll wonder what they should have done differently, caught earlier. And they'll stand near the coffee machine muttering about incurable diseases, sounding too professional, and then sneak home and bury their faces in their pillows.

For doctors death is the ultimate enemy. Death is not the end result of all life. Death is an unnatural force that steals promising patients away in the dark of night. Death is messy and abrupt. Death is not to be talked about. (Death might show up if you call its name too loud.) Our fears of death only remind the doctor of the ocean of knowledge he never learned or long ago forgot. Death reminds him of the futility of his efforts and his own eventual demise. And isn't his work hard enough without being reminded of these dreadful things?

Saul was smaller than I expected. He wore a white lab coat that nearly reached the floor, his gray hair surrounding a bald spot. He was different from any physician I'd ever met, he had presence. The first time we met, he strode into the room and immediately came to where I was sitting and put his hand on my shoulder. His hand felt large and heavy for such a small man. "I am Dr. Rosenberg," he told me.

I knew who he was. I'd done my homework. I'd used my skills as a graduate student researcher to pore over the literature on Hodgkin's disease. I'd phoned physicians in hospitals across the country and insisted on speaking to them, tapping an assertiveness that only comes from fear of death. My research and their words were consistent. "Rosenberg is world class."

When I relapsed the second time it was the September before Terry and I were scheduled to be married. I'd survived the bone marrow transplant for nothing. My first instinct was to avoid doctors and enjoy life until I died, but then I grew curious. Just like the first time I read the end of *Romeo and Juliet*, I wondered, Is it really over? There were hints. An oncologist who knew Terry had cornered her in the hall. "Dan has one last chance," he'd whispered.

Everywhere Saul went a trail of residents followed. They had the look of scared mice. Eager. Nervous. And when he laid hands on me, I knew he was the man. He was the only person who found my tumors faster than I could. His hands were strong and forceful but also glided with precision. Most physicians and nurses had too soft a touch and never really found what I'd found long before them: those hard, smooth beans forged from heavy tire rubber.

Eventually he had all of the information. He had every scan I had ever taken, each chemotherapeutic agent I'd ingested, every rad of radiation documented. A fellow had pored over each piece of information and summarized it for him in a neat three-page document. He'd put his hands on my neck and under my arms and around my groin searching for cancer. He came into our room and put his hands on my shoulders. He looked into my face. "I don't think I can cure you," he said, "but I'm going to try."

I turned those words over and over again, searching for every nuance of meaning. His pessimism frightened me. His willingness to try was thrilling.

We went back to Gainesville and stayed one month before moving out to Stanford. Terry told Saul we had to pack, and there was something else we needed to do.

Against Advice

My chest fills with the sound of soft mallets on steel drums, the calypso. Jamaican voices weave a blanket of melodies around us. Terry's face is lit; she smiles at me as she spins with her father. If I listen carefully I can hear another rhythm below the drums; it's the sound of Sunday shoes tapping on the outdoor wooden floor.

Behind the dancing mass of friends and relatives there's a back-drop of hundreds of dreaming spires, flower stalks, each with a blue face and brown eye. I spin and sway, the spires make a blue curtain. I giggle at them and throw my head toward a cloudless evening sky. The smell of Chinese spring rolls comes and goes, and I stop for a moment. Now a pleasant young face offers me a nibblet from the sea, baked inside a flour casement, each morsel leaning against the next on a silver plate that glints in the candle-light. I've given up trying to remember it all. Trying to stay aware of each moment of our wedding. Faces familiar from childhood and adolescence are mingled with those of adulthood; they come and wish me well and disappear.

Soon Terry and I will sequester ourselves in the back suite. With the last sweat of the day we'll consummate this marriage.

For one month I was separated from the normal ebb and flow of life in the bone marrow transplant unit. There were no panty hose or toothpaste commercials, no bills or graduate student deadlines. I didn't change any flat tires, or answer any urgent patient calls. Most of my time in the transplant unit I lived in a drug-induced fog. But there were rare moments of clarity, when fog lifted and the air was clean. During one of those respites I thought of Terry and a home, and children.

I figured out once that Terry had closely cared for two hundred patients who had died. When we first dated, I noticed that around her house there were pictures of her with smiling bald faces, her vamping and giggling captured on Kodak paper.

When I relapsed the warnings from her friends, silent for so long, came on stronger than ever. Stern. Pleading. "Oh Terry, what are you doing?" and "It's not your responsibility to save him"

and "You know where he's headed." One colleague listed the
patients with Hodgkin's whom they had both known who had
died, Jodi's name among them. Later Terry would tell me that she
had tried not to listen to him, but sometimes, walking from her
car into the hospital, or surveying breads at the supermarket, she
would see the patients' faces—and the faces of their parents and
children, husbands and wives.

I got down on my knees four months after the transplant, and a
year before we learned of my second relapse. During a comfortable dinner I walked to her side of the table, dropped to a knee,
and held her hand. We'd never spoken about marriage. We didn't
joke about it, there was no teasing, it was never mentioned. Looking up at her I waited for some response. "You're kidding, right?"
she asked. I showed her the ring. No joke. And with quiet certainty
she looked through me and whispered, "I'll marry you. Yes. Yes.
Yes."

Autumn weddings in Gainesville are not easy to plan. In some corners of the world stadiums are rocked by soccer. Fans have been
known to destroy bleachers and riot if something goes awry on the
field. Closer to home there are towns where the name of every
high-school basketball player is known. Gainesville, though, bows
down only to the pigskin. On Gator home-game weekends
Gainesville swells like a mosquito at a reunion picnic. The roads
clog with recreational vehicles painted a nausea-inducing bright
orange and blue, and every hotel and motel bed is happily claimed
for double the normal price. GO GATOR T-shirts and banners and
baseball caps adorn both young and old.

    It's not a good time to have a wedding, so we planned the
ceremony for the first weekend in November. An away-game

day. We were safe! We found a bed-and-breakfast called Hurlong, an old Southern mansion located in Micanopy, a small town south of Gainesville that claims to be the first incorporated town in America. It was a perfect site. It had Ionic columns supporting a dignified overhang. A brick walk leading up to the house, perfect for a processional. A sitting porch, where a brass quintet could use the house to echo the melodies my brother wrote for us. And all surrounded by a wide lawn enclosed by short hedges where our guests could watch us exchange the vows we'd written ourselves.

We made arrangements. Food. A dance floor. Flowers. Cake. The brass quintet and a calypso band. A few weeks before the wedding, Sonny, the proprietor of the bed-and-breakfast, phoned. I listened to his slow Southern pace. "Bad news, I'm afraid, your wedding is the same day as the annual Micanopy Folk Art Festival. I've tried talking to the council, but it's no use, the street'll be blocked off with two hundred tables. They'll be selling all sorts of crafts. The good news is I got 'em to skip the accordion competition, but I'm afraid that's all I can do. Hope y'all will still come."

We balked initially, but then considered the invitations that had already been sent out, the plane reservations that had already been made, the band and hors d'oeuvres already arranged for. And maybe also the knowledge that time was limited.

I watched Terry walk down the aisle. When the brass quintet started the wedding processional, Micanopy paused. The crowd stopped surveying clay wind chimes and watercolors, silver earrings and fried dough, and gathered along the short hedges of the mansion to watch. Hundreds of faces. When the music ended, the street was silent. I could hear birds, and a light breeze fluttered the canopy set up in case of rain. Terry nuzzled in next to me and took my hand. I looked from her out over the massive gathering, and I couldn't be sure, but it felt as if the world was holding its breath for us.

A Last Will

"Sperm, sperm, sperm," said the lawyer. I watched him bang a Ticonderoga Adirondack #2 pencil against his head. He tapped it furiously and it left a little red welt just above his brow. The brass eraser head glinted and left an orange trail in the office's afternoon light. The attorney had a thick mustache that was longer on one side than the other. Red and gray whiskers bowed over his upper lip from beneath his nose. He looked at the ceiling while the pencil tapped away. "Wha'd'ya suppose the appropriate measurement for sperm is? They don't count 'em, do they?" he said. I was about to answer but realized he was thinking out loud. "Nah, they probably do it in milliliters, right?" He looked at me, pointed at me with the pencil and lowered his voice. "This is important." The pencil tip pointed at me, bobbing in midair. "We don't want anyone else trying to claim your sperm."

I agreed. I tried to imagine a stranger standing in court, asking for the right to have my sperm. "Your Honor, I think I should have the remaining sperm. After all, Teresa Shapiro only has a legal right to twenty milliliters of it . . ."

The pencil hovered, waiting. I offered, "I think the sperm are kept in vials. Maybe we should just say 'seventeen vials.'" He looked at me.

"That's good. That's very good. That'll work," he said and scratched notes furiously. "I don't get many kids in here doing wills, you involved in something shady? You need some help?"

When I said no he squinted at me. "You got some kind of disease, huh?" I told him I did. "Tough luck, kid."

Two days earlier, on a Saturday morning, Terry'd approached me in the kitchen. I was groggily pulling eggs from the refrigerator when she came up behind me and snuggled her head between my shoulder blades, her arms wrapped around my chest. "Honey," she started. "I want to have your children." I suggested that I'd be happy to go back upstairs and . . . but her voice carried a different tone. "No, I mean I want to have your children, even if Stanford doesn't work out." *If I die.* She let go and I got a bowl. I broke the eggs into the bowl and slowly stirred, staring into the swirling mass. She took the fork from me and whipped the eggs quickly, the sound of the metal clinking against the side of the bowl punctuating her question. "I want to raise your children. I know this. I don't know if I'd ever want another man in my life, but I do want to raise little Daniels." She was stirring too fast. I stopped her arm for a second. "I need to think about this one."

After breakfast I went for a drive. Alone. Drove east to 75, got on, and headed south. The road was clear, it was a Saturday, and I pressed the car past the speed limit. *Can I justify inviting my child into the world without me here to look after it? What happens to children born without fathers? Isn't that the ultimate in carelessness?* I knew of my mother's anguish, the way she'd idealized her father, missed him desperately, and sometimes hated him for not living.

But what about Terry? Didn't she have a right? Wouldn't I want her to raise my children? I took the Archer Road exit and headed back into town to Shands Hospital. I found my favorite cubicle in the medical school library and buried myself in the literature. I looked for research studies on children and resilience. I was surprised by what I found. The studies suggested that children raised by at least one devoted and caring adult were usually

resilient. They coped well with challenges and were able to
develop relationships even under horrible circumstances.

I tried to imagine being raised by Terry. I'd seen her around
children on the bone marrow transplant unit. They loved her. She
talked straight with them, was physical and affectionate, could set
limits and be playful. She had Indiana common sense.

As I walked out of the library I saw a woman leading a little
girl, maybe three years old, through the door. The mother looked
straight ahead, pushing open the glass doors while the girl caught
my eye, stared at me, bronze ringlets curled around her mouth.
She smiled and then her mother lifted her up into her arms and
they were gone.

On Monday I called the sperm bank and asked what I needed to
do to put Terry's name on my sperm.

"Get a lawyer," the voice told me.

I, Daniel Edward Shapiro, a resident of Gainesville, Alachua
County, State of Florida, being of sound and disposing mind and
memory, do hereby declare this to be my Last Will and Testament,
hereby revoking and annulling all other Wills and Codicils made
by me at any time heretofore. To my wife, Teresa Shapiro, I give,
devise, and bequeath the following: seventeen vials of sperm. . . .

Sergio's Very First and Only Free Haircut

"You come to see Sergio, you come to the best, eh?" Sergio said. He patted his chair and bowed slightly. "You come a-sit in my chair and let me a-make magic with your hair again." I smiled at him and sat in the chair, watched him in the mirror. "I haven't a-seen you in a few months, you-a been seeing someone else?" I shook my head. Sergio was dressed all in white—white slacks, a white button-down shirt and a white silk tie. His wing-tips were red. Both of his pinkies had hot-red fingernail polish. His hair was gelled and combed back. I thought he was in his early forties.

Sergio was the first person who ever cut my hair while standing far away. He'd stand, one hand on a hip, the other in midair with the scissors. Then he'd flick his wrist toward my head and locks of my hair would fall on the floor. I could always hear the scissors flicking open and shut with a whisk. He never used one hand to hold the hair and the other to cut. Sergio was strictly a one-handed stylist.

He spun me toward the mirror. "People say to me, 'Sergio, a-Sergio, a-Sergio, how did you get to be a-so good at a-hair? Where did you-a come from that you are a-so good at a-cutting hair?' I say I was a-born in Florence, I was a-born with a blow-dryer in my hands and I grabbed the doctor's scalpel and a-did his hair before I went home with my a-mama, Godresthersoul."

"It's good to see you, Sergio." I got the words in before he continued.

"So-a you still with your a-beautiful new wife? How-a come she don't a-let me cut her hair?" he asked, combing.

I thought for a moment. "I'm too afraid if she meets you she'll never want to be with me again, Sergio."

He laughed. "Now-a, you make a-fun of Sergio, heh? You think it's-a funny to keep me from-a my destiny? I make her very beautiful. You won't wanna do nothing but be with her after I do her-a hair, yes?"

Sergio stood away from me and surveyed me as if he were a painter. "So, enough a-chatter, you-a talk too much." I watched him in the mirror. He reached forward with one hand and held the end of my hair below my neck. "What magic am I a-working today?"

I braced myself. "Sergio, I need you to cut it all off," I said.

There was a pause. Sergio squinted at me and then smiled wide. "That's a-very funny. You joke with Sergio, heh? You think that's a-funny, eh? Maybe I a-show you, maybe I a-go ahead and a-cut it all off, then you laugh, heh, make you look like a-Kojak, ha-ha!" Sergio pointed at me, emphasizing that the joke would be on me.

I said quietly, "I mean it, Sergio. That's what I want. Cut it all off. We're leaving for California tomorrow so I can get more chemo. I don't want it falling out slowly and getting all over everything."

Sergio paused, his hand still holding the ends of my hair. "You-a sick again?"

I nodded. He squinted again.

We looked at each other. I said it again. "Cut it all off. I want to be smooth when I leave here." I rubbed my head as if to show him what I wanted.

Sergio looked at me in the mirror, moved closer to me. He put a hand on my cheek and whispered without even a trace of the Italian accent, "You know, I lost my Michael to the gay disease. I'm so sorry you're sick again. I'll take care of you." Sergio cleared his throat, opened a drawer and lifted out his electric razor. Plugged it in. He turned it on and seemed startled by its insistent buzz.

He held the buzzing razor with one hand and studied it for a moment, running his other hand through my hair. Then his open hand settled on my ear and he pressed me gently into his chest while he started to shear, ever so slowly, as if he were painting a masterpiece with a tiny paintbrush, stroke by stroke. As the first locks fell on my shoulders I felt myself well up—*Here we go again*—and when I looked at Sergio in the mirror his eyes were closed; he was moving the razor with slow strokes and bobbing his head almost imperceptibly, as if to a dirge only he could hear. I sat quietly, pressed into his warm chest, feeling my hair descend like light rain.

When he was done I was bald. Just as he was finishing, another patron sat down in the waiting area and Sergio suddenly stood back, looking away from me, and said loudly, "There, you-a bastard, next time you-a insult me I'll shave-a off your eyebrows too. Now a-get ah out of here! I donna want-a none of your a-dirty money, neither." I smiled at him and stood up. Rubbed my bald head. I turned and headed out of the salon. When I looked back at Sergio, he mouthed, "Godspeed, sweetie," and was holding his hands together in prayer like a mother.

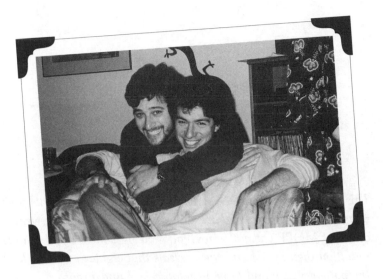

Part Five

Salvage

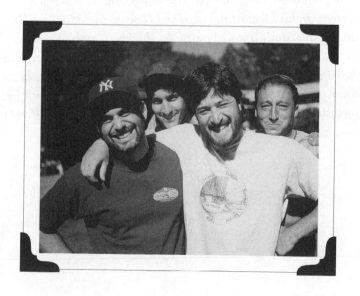

Dictated Chart Note

7/91

This is an unfortunate 24-year-old white male who presents with relapsed stage II-B Hodgkin's disease. In 1987 he underwent 6 cycles of MOPP chemotherapy, followed by 2400 cGy of mantle radiation therapy. Chart review reveals that eighteen months later the patient was found to be in relapse and underwent an autologous bone marrow transplant. He recently presented, one year and one month following his transplant, with a new right supraclavicular node. This node was biopsied and was consistent with recurrent nodular sclerosing Hodgkin's disease. Following complete evaluation performed here, the patient was found to have a possible increase in his Mediastinal mass on CT scan. In addition, a lymphangiogram study showed possible shoddy lymph nodes in the inguinal area. Patient is newly married. He and wife have relocated here from Gainesville for his chemotherapy and radiation. In summary, the patient presents following a second relapse with likely metastatic disease for salvage chemotherapy with a final attempt to cure his disease.

JOSHUA SOKOL, M.D.
Stanford Medical Center

Spirit Doctors

Hey thanks. Bleary-eyed resident with short hair and a starched collar, pissed off at four A.M. 'cause the coffeepot's empty and you'll only get ten minutes before you have to come into my room 'cause I've spiked another damned fever and I'm complaining about my Hickman catheter again. Thanks for sitting down when you came in. Thanks for taking the time to listen before you grabbed for the catheter.

Hey you, the nurse who told me yesterday your son is failing out of school — "What's with kids these days?" — with your tall hair and all those pins from hospitals around the country on your lapel. You smiled and stroked my arm.

Hey you. Big man. Standing awkward at the end of my bed with tools on your belt. Shifting your weight like you did when your mom told you not to touch anything at the curio store. You told me three times you were there to check the thermometer 'cause I'd complained and you knew how tough it was to be cold when you're feeling sick. You apologized for the intrusion, said it slow, *in-true-sion*. You asked me if it was a good time. You could come back if I wanted to sleep now. Thanks.

Hey thanks. Big woman with yellow eyes and thick hands who pushed my wheelchair and hummed "Danny Boy."

Hey radiology tech with a faded blue tattoo on the webbing between your thumb and pointer who helped me pull off my T-shirt. "That's okay, my man. No apologies needed. Gonna take good care of you, I'm the best," you said, and for a minute I didn't worry that the X ray might get lost or not come out.

Hey thanks. Oncology fellow who let me talk about graduate school at two A.M. when I couldn't sleep from the chemotherapy. You hung in my doorway like a kid hanging on jungle bars, and asked me questions about my research like a student might, and let me blather on as if I had something to contribute.

Thanks. Old voice who answered the phone when I dialed the operator. Not sure how to locate someone at the pharmacy to ask them to hold my prescriptions. You took the time to ask me questions. A voice of a seasoned grandmother who'd raised six kids by herself. You figured out who I might need to call. Didn't just give me the number but ran interference for me. Called and made sure they were there. You saved me a trip on a feverish day. Thanks.

And you. Old lady in a faded pink smock, gray eyebrows and a tall black wig who gave me a newspaper in the morning and told me it was cold outside. "Brrrrr," you said and lifted your shoulders, pretending to shiver.

Hey thanks. You carrying the Bibles around with those callused hands, wearing the collar and the rolled-up sleeves. It's not my speed, but I appreciated how kind and honest you were. No pretense and no trying to convert me. Just a polite offer.

And you. The girl with thin elbows and a Cuban way of trilling your r's, who brings the trays of food I don't eat these days. Your brown smooth skin. You shake your head at me and tell me I need to eat if I'm going to get strong, even though you don't blame me 'cause you think the food is all overcooked. You make me smile.

Sometimes, when my body has forgotten how to regulate its temperature and the world has grown cold. When I don't recognize my puffy, bald reflection. When I notice the hair on my arms is gone and my veins are just dry winter branches. Sometimes there are fleeting thoughts. *I'm already gone. It's already over. Why not stop fighting?* And then one of you enters my room and laughs with me, or flirts, or tells me about a good movie. And I'm back. I'm still alive. And I'm gonna kick this thing.

Enlightenment Under Pressure

Here's to the acoustic guitar. A callused finger strumming blue-grass folk. The stuff I put in my ears during chemotherapy infusions. Melodies of struggle, lost loves and barroom brawls, work battles and motel loneliness. I'd never found folk blues comforting before. But from the middle of the first round of chemotherapy on, I never hooked up for chemotherapy without a similar infusion of acoustic therapy. James Taylor singing about kicking heroin or Jim Croce's junkyard dogs, Bonnie Raitt's setting a lover straight or Carole King's urban rooftop blues.

Here's to the Cajun chef. Daytime television cook. A man who can turn chopping an onion (pronounced *on-YAN*) into a festival. A flannel-shirted, suspendered soul who talks to his vegetables: "Don't you, ah, make a fool of me on television, Mr. Tomato," and "'Scuse me, Mr. Sweet Red Pepper, I'm gonna put you over here out of the way. You won't mind, huh?" I smiled along with him for hours, watching his spices and vegetables and sauces swirl together into culinary delights in wooden bowls while the bags of medicine and poison emptied into my hand.

Here's to the public-television painter of oil landscapes. A kind man with Brillo hair. I'd never watched him before chemotherapy. But suddenly I found him enchanting. The way he used a putty knife to make mountaintops, and a fluffy brush to make bushes, and the quick way he turned his wrist while mixing white and gray paint to make an ice-covered river. "Be brave," he said once, dabbing a rag to form clouds. "There's no mistakes here. Anything you do is delightful." And I smiled. What a wonderful way to teach people, huddled in front of their televisions, to free themselves enough to release their own art.

Health psychologists rely heavily on relaxation and distraction. Distraction to a psychologist is the act of engaging in something absorbing to avoid thinking about the important, horrible thing that's happening simultaneously. The problem with psychologists' distraction is that it assumes that life stops during horrible things, that it's impossible to continue living fully during challenges. Over time, I developed a different philosophy, that of enlightenment under pressure. It's still possible to enjoy life's offerings, even in the face of physical and psychological challenge. Life doesn't stop when something horrible happens. Even chemotherapy can't eclipse James Taylor's smooth tenor, the Cajun chef's playful bantering with a parsnip, and the magic of a putty knife on stretched canvas.

Coach Douglas

Wrestling season was in the winter, but the gym was hot. Coach Douglas kept it at eighty degrees to help us lose weight and to startle opposing teams when they visited. Heat hissed and knocked out of peeling brown pipes that ran behind the closed bleachers. The gym had high frosted windows and during the first thirty minutes of practice there was still faint sunlight streaming in, gold and blue, through the glass. Then the light faded and we grabbed and spun under fluorescent lamps high on the gym ceiling.

Bloomfield High was a midsized public high school in northern Connecticut with about nine hundred students, black, white, Hispanic, and Asian. The football team was a statewide contender year after year and attracted most of the small athletic budget. Not so the wrestling team. Before every practice we unrolled three hard mats that were thirty years old. When we were thrown or flipped the mats came up to meet us, hard and fast.

I don't think Coach Douglas would remember me. There were quite a few students, quite a few wrestlers. But I would remember him, even without wrestling. I was in his ninth-grade history class. He was the first and only teacher I had during my education who administered "A or F" tests. If we didn't earn 90 percent, we failed. And if a student didn't earn an A in history, Mr. Douglas would make the student bring his report card to class and tape it to his chest every day for a week.

My first wrestling practice was startling. First we ran three miles. Then Mr. Douglas gathered everyone on the ancient mats and paired experienced wrestlers with new ones. He yelled out, "Riding drills," and blew a whistle. Mike Stanavicius, a team captain, was partnered with me. Stanavicius quickly threw me to the mat on my stomach and got on top of me. He whispered in my ear, "Get up, ya faggot." I pushed myself up and he pulled my arms from under me. I groaned. "Whassa matter, faggot?" he whispered. I pushed again and he pulled my arms again. My face was turned sideways, pressed hard into the thick rubber mat. "Ya better be tougher than this, Shapiro."

Rage. I pushed up abruptly and tried to spin into him, but he was faster and managed to stay behind me. I tried to escape by bolting forward, but he had my wrists before I could kneel and I was back, facedown. I groaned and writhed. Managed to lift again, this time his weight and mine—TRIUMPH!?—but he kicked my legs out from under me and I was down again. My teeth gritted together. I spun. I lifted. I grabbed. But each time he was faster and stronger, his voice unwavering in my ear. "Z'at all you got, Shapiro?" No. No. More spinning. More lifting. More rolling and grabbing. My arms shook and I wanted to surrender as tears welled in my eyes.

I heard the whistle blow and Stanavicius stood up. I didn't realize I was supposed to stand. I lingered on the mat, my arms shaking, wiping the rage from my eyes. Suddenly Coach Douglas's face was next to mine. I could see each shaven whisker on his cheek. He was insistent. "You're okay, get up."

I wanted to quit. Right then. Walk off. Other kids did. But I didn't. And I wanted to the next week and the one after that. I hated the heat. I hated the splinters in my fingers from climbing ropes and the way my lungs grabbed for air after the windsprints. I hated the three-mile runs around the gym, sixty laps, before practice, and the water fountain filled with spit. I hated getting beaten up by Stanavicius, the way he used his forearms to choke off the air while he whispered, "Faggot." I hated being too scared to shower in a place where other kids had been held down and shaved of all their pubic hair. I hated waiting for my mother outside after practice, unshowered, sweat turning cold on my chest and legs.

But more than any of it, I hated Coach Douglas. I hated the way he used our ethnicities to motivate us. "You know, Shapiro," he said, his arm wrapped around my head, "the Israelis are the toughest fighters in the world—you could learn from them." Then I heard him tell Mike Stanavicius that the Lithuanians were the toughest fighters in the world. And Fran Marino about the Italians and Paul Kennedy about the Irish. I hated the way he pitted us against one another, told us how each man should watch the others for "dogging it," deliberate cheating, not working out hard. I hated how I felt around him, how I studied his face for any sign of acceptance or praise. The way he'd lean over me if I took an extra second to get up after being pinned. "You're okay. Get up." I hated his questions: "Do you have the tenacity to endure?" and "Are you willing to fight through your exhaustion?" and "Are you tougher than the other man?"

Eventually the weeks passed. I won a varsity jacket and held the spot, despite staring at the ceiling fans during most matches while some other boy's father applauded. I loved the wrestling jacket and wore it constantly, trying not to think about why I was proud of a jacket that represented a sport I didn't enjoy.

Ten years later I found my knees pressing on bathroom tile, wrestling's starting position. I was two months into salvage chemotherapy, wearing down. I'd had shingles and mouth sores and had lost twenty-five pounds. While looking at the porcelain rim after releasing everything in my stomach, a thought occurred to me: *This is terrible.* It led to *Why me?* and more. I was just getting momentum, the litany swirling together into a serious pity fest, when I heard that annoying gravelly, Midwestern voice: "You're okay. Get up."

Hope Junkie's Lament

I don't want much. You know I'm not greedy. I just want a little taste today. Come on. Hook me up. Help me out here.

I know how you look at me. Why you keep your distance. To you I'm just another twitching junkie. Steel-burned veins and long eyes. Tattered. Tired. Strung out. You know the truth about me. I can hide it from everyone but you, huh? You know I've been sticking hope in my veins. I jam it in, snort it, snuff it, drink it. I rub it on my chest. You know I need it. You know I deserve it. The hunger is constant. Shit, you're the only dealer I trust, so don't turn away from me today, please.

You know, it's partially your fault. You got me started. You hooked me up for free at the very beginning when you said, "The bad news is it's cancer, but the good news is it's curable." From then on you had me. I hang on every drop you send my way now.

You know, Doc, sometimes I see the clean faces in the waiting rooms and I can't stand them. The ones who know they're dying and don't need the hope anymore. They can let it go. No more torture, wondering if they're going to live. Or not. They know. They can say their good-byes and live fully until the end. They've given up the drug, kicked the habit.

And the others. The ones I really hate. With their above-the-fray smugness. The ones who were never in danger. They reek of that calmness that only comes with the certainty that they'll live no matter what happens today. They don't need the hope. Never did. I catch their glances, their politeness, and their "Oh, take my seat, you need it more" bullshit.

I need you to help me out. I haven't slept and I got that fire restlessness in my belly, as if there's somewhere I have to go, but we both know there's nowhere. You know, I don't have a problem, I could stop if I wanted to, I could acknowledge how bad it all is. Just face the facts, but I don't want to. It's the only high left for me.

You know, Doc, I can admit it. I love hope. I fucking love it. When I'm high on hope it's the only time I find relief. Nothing can touch me when I'm floating in it. Not the nausea, the numb fingers and toes, or my burned-out insides. Not your bureaucracy with insurance letters and claim forms. Not the sad looks from Terry. It's all gone when I'm high on hope.

But the highs end faster these days. I seem to need more and more to keep me going. You didn't tell me this would happen.

You gave me no warning, man. It used to be that a tiny droplet of hope from you could coast me for a month. Just a little word, *progress* or *encouraging*, could send me into the ether. No more. Now each sign of my worsening condition cleans the hope out faster. And then there's another discouraging sign and another and another and pretty soon I'm totally strung out and desperate to come in here and see you again, even though I just left. Like today I noticed it took extra work to open a door and then just a few minutes later your nurse told me I've lost even more weight. . . .

Don't look at me that way, Doc, I'm not telling you this to make you think I need something huge here. I just want a little taste. That's all. Just a nip of what you've got, Doc. Hook me up. Tell me it's looking better. Look me in the eyes and tell me *I'm* getting better. Tell me all this shit is worth it. Come on, Doc. You know I'm good for it, don't you?

Okay, hold on now. I hear you, I hear you. I'm not greedy. Don't turn away from me. Please. Come on, we've known each other awhile now, haven't we? And I can still make you laugh. That's worth something.

How 'bout this. Just give me a pat. Yeah. How 'bout just a little pat on the shoulder. And maybe a smile and a "You're doing fine." That's all I'm asking for. That's not much, huh? Come on, Doc. Hook me up. Hook me up.

Hail to the Prince

I am sword fighting in a barren field of rocks. Nearby a medieval carriage rests. Inside, behind a plush purple curtain, a mysterious prince watches. The landscape is cold and hostile. A light wind blows snowy powder into my face. The air feels dry. I glance down and notice that I'm wearing plaid pajama bottoms with red feet. The feet are the kind with gray plastic on the bottom and cotton on the top. I'm bare-chested. I'm rather proud of my pajamas. My opponent wears heavy black armor from head to toe, including a hockey mask and a helmet. His silver eyes glare angrily behind angled eye slits.

My opponent thrusts with grace despite the weight of his huge polished sword. Effortlessly, he slices the air near my head. It suddenly occurs to me that he is trying to kill me. I have to do something. I dodge and counterattack, lunging forward, but I am inanely slow and awkward. It seems to take decades for me to get my hands to respond. My weapon shakes clumsily and I hold on with both hands as if I'm clutching a galleon oar instead of a sword. I swing blindly, grunting with the effort, and miss him completely. He slides closer. I can hear his calm breathing. His sword starts behind him and swings swiftly toward my neck. I'm about to die.

I'm suddenly awake. Pain shoots through my spine, across my back, and down my arms. Terry sleeps soundly nearby. The morning sun has not risen. Our room is dark save for a bright digital clock which casts a red glow on everything. What's happening? The covers are around my ankles and I'm all twisted around.

Agony. Searing pain. It's excruciating and relentless. As the fog clears from the dream, a fear supplements the pain. A fierce, primal anxiety. What is this pain from? *Take a moment, clear your head, and take stock.* The anguish seems to be radiating from my hips. *Perhaps it's nothing. Perhaps I was just sleeping funny. That must be it. That silly dream got me all bunched up. Pajamas with feet on them. How absurd. I'll take a few deep, calm breaths and think of something else. Maybe I'll take a shower. Yes, a shower will take the kinks out. A fine idea. Then maybe a short walk while watching the sunrise.* I move a little, rocking my hips in bed and swiveling my torso. Every slight movement initiates a new round of spinal writhing and screeching. Pain blares a siren. This pain is not the product of sleeping funny. Something is very wrong.

The cancer has spread to my bones. I must have bone metastases. I'm dying. I'm finished. There's nothing else it could be. I haven't exercised, I haven't pulled any muscles, I've never had arthritis or any muscular disorders. The dream was a warning. Once Hodgkin's attacks the bone, Hodgkin's patients are finished. Death is near. I can almost smell it. I wake Terry and tell her that I have strange pains in my spine. She's calming. We should wait until the clinic opens. Good thinking. I don't want to be one of the millions in the emergency room. We'll wait.

I walk, hunched over, into the bathroom and wash up. It's hard to draw a breath. Terry rises sleepily and starts her morning rituals. I sit at the kitchen table, but no position seems comfortable. I have one medical thing I need to do before we leave. I'm supposed to give myself a growth factor shot. Growth factors, which stimulate bone marrow to produce cells, are new. During my first treatment, and then again during the bone marrow transplant, growth factors did not exist. I've managed to live long enough to see this new invention, which might have saved my life. I can receive higher doses of chemotherapy now with growth factors because my white blood cells rebound so quickly. But now that I've relapsed, perhaps the growth factors will also stimulate the cancer cells? I try to remember how growth factors work, but my mind is sluggish. I'm not sure I should take the shot and I don't. Besides, what difference will the growth factors make now that cancer has spread to my bones? I'll stop all of this chemotherapy nonsense the minute it's confirmed.

The drive to the hospital takes forever. It's still impossible to find a comfortable position. Each slight bump in the road reverberates up my spine. I haven't told Terry my suspicion about the bone metastases. I don't want to trouble her. I count the mile post signs and watch the other drivers in the rush-hour traffic.

Doubled over in the waiting room of the clinic, still in acute pain, I rehearse how Saul, a physician I have come to worship, will tell me the bad news. After asking me a bunch of questions, he will put his hand on my shoulder and tell me he wants to get some tests done, a CAT scan, maybe a gallium scan. I will ask why he wants the tests and he will tell me, because he's never hedged before, "I think the Hodgkin's may have spread to your bones," and Terry will bite her lower lip and breathe too fast while trying to look calm, as if everything is going to work out all right. I'll say, "I'm done, then, no more treatment," and he'll say, "I understand, but we do have some palliative weapons in our arsenal," and I will say, "No. No more. It's time to go home," and we'll shake hands. Very dignified. I hope I don't dissociate. I hate that.

A young patient sits near me who still has his hair. His cheeks have a rosy glow, he's been outside. He clutches a rolled-up magazine too tight—maybe this is his first treatment? I envy him.

I am invited into an examining room and I wait for Saul. I steel myself for the news I am about to hear and try to stay focused. I feel my mind shutting down and I fight it. *Be dignified.* Eventually, Saul appears, with a gaggle of residents and fellows behind him. They fill the room. Two of them have been joking in the hall, but they quickly calm themselves when they step into the room. Serious. Saul begins to introduce the cast of characters. Then he asks why I've come in. I describe the pain. I point at my hips and my spine while gesticulating to emphasize how severe it is. I use the words *stabbing* and *darting*. Saul listens patiently and nods his head slowly, looking stern. I know he's about to ask me to undergo extensive testing to determine the extent of bone involvement. But I don't want anything else. I'm done with this place, the treatment. I want to go home. But Saul says nothing. He leans back away from me and looks at the wall behind me. I turn around to see what he's looking at. There's a small crack in the wall. "Any other symptoms or side effects?" he asks me. I turn back around. "Uh, no," I say. He asks one of the young physicians standing next to him, "Tell me his dosage of Neupogen." The young doctor studies a folder in his hand and turns a few pages. "Uh, four hundred eighty mics per day," he says. Saul puts his hand on my shoulder. *Here it comes.* I fight to stay focused. "Daniel, bone pain, the kind of pain you describe, is a common side effect of growth factors, the Neupogen. It's a sign that your marrow is working hard and effectively. Your white blood cell count is very high. It's common. Dr. Edwards, be so kind as to prescribe some Vicodin for our boy here, and let's hold his growth factor for now." And then to me: "The Vicodin should ease your pain. Anything else?" Dr. Edwards whips out a prescription pad and scratches away, balancing it on a colleague's back. Meanwhile Saul and the rest of the gaggle head out of the room.

I'm not dying? I rock my hips and notice that suddenly the pain doesn't seem so severe. It's even a little entertaining. "Hey, I'm the Tin Man! Oil me!" Terry rubs my bald head and laughs.

As Saul goes through the door, just for a moment, the back of his head is illuminated. Hair surrounds his bald spot which shines in the light. He looks as if he's wearing a crown. Then I realize, Saul is the prince. The prince of Stanford. Hail to the prince. Hail!

Hope

Before moving to California to get the last treatment, I worked on a locked inpatient psychiatry unit at Shands Hospital where my job was to run groups. I met Joe there, a patient in his early sixties. He was thin and gaunt, hunched forward, and though he shaved every day, he had a permanent dark streak of stubble across his cheeks and chin. His voice was gruff and cigarette low. In group he kept his hands folded over his chest and he turned himself to one side, as if he wasn't really listening.

Joe was admitted to the locked ward after a suicide attempt. He'd been found in his truck in his garage, carbon monoxide leaking out from under the door. When his brother arrived, intent on returning tools he'd borrowed before a fight with Joe, he saw the thick rolls of smoke. He lifted the door and dragged his older brother out to the driveway, the fumes of exhaust and whiskey heavy on Joe's clothing.

During his first week Joe said nothing in the daily group. He occasionally rolled his eyes in response to other patients, but when I or my coleader pressed him to participate, he just shook his head. On the unit he carried himself with authority, as if he was used to institutions, but he kept the staff at arm's length. His chart told an incomplete story. Joe had been in eight hospitals in the previous four years with no history of problems before that. *What happened four years ago? Maybe he lost a job or a wife,* I thought. It's not unusual for older men to bounce into hospitals when they're suddenly isolated or lose the roles that have given them purpose.

On the seventh day after Joe's admission, a younger man, in his forties, was admitted to the unit after crashing his car. His family thought it was a suicide attempt and had him hospitalized. The newcomer chatted constantly, dominating the group. He had opinions about everything and commented after anyone spoke. He started each sentence with, "Well, if it were me, I would . . . ," and out would come advice, most of it drivel. At first Joe seemed disinterested as usual. But over the course of the session he began to squirm in his seat until he seemed ready to burst.

One of the patients asked the young man why he was in the hospital. He responded that it was a mistake, that his car had malfunctioned and his crazy family had admitted him against his will.

"They're the ones that ought to be in here, know what I mean?" he said. Joe burst. His powerful low voice caught the entire group by surprise. "You're full of shit," he started, raising a pointed finger at the younger man. "You're in here same as me. You tried to off yourself with your car. You drink, huh?"

The younger man swallowed and bobbed his head back on his shoulders, like a boy afraid of being struck. He defended himself quietly. "I have a few, but I control it —"

"BULLSHIT!" Joe yelled. "Bullshit, bullshit, bullshit, you're a fucking alcoholic, same as me. Tellin' everyone their business. Bullshit." Joe dropped his finger and crossed his arms over himself again. His eyes didn't leave the younger man.

Joe's voice had shocked me. I looked back at the younger man. His eyebrows were tight and he was studying his sneakers. I could see a thick blotch of red-hot skin on his neck. He was totally silent for the first time. When I looked around the group, I saw the other members were smiling. Joe was a hero.

From then on, Joe talked in group. The group wanted to know everything about him and with each session we heard a little more of his story. His wife had died fifteen years before. He'd missed her at first but had done okay. He'd worked as a printer his entire life, right up until his admission. He'd been an alcoholic since returning from the Korean War, but until four years ago, his drinking hadn't dominated his life. Then he spun out of control. He wouldn't tell us what happened. "I don't want to talk about it," he said.

The days passed. Joe started participating in every part of the treatment process; he slept and ate well, he had strong concentration, and he even seemed to be nurturing some of the other patients. It was time for him to leave. He'd be discharged to outpatient treatment.

At his last group he said good-bye to everyone. He said he didn't want to talk, but the group pressed him as if they were journalists, peppering him with questions about what had happened four years before. He dodged and weaved, but eventually one of the patients he'd been helping stopped him.

"Joe, come on. I've told you everything. What happened?"

Joe looked at me and then rubbed the bridge of his nose. He squeezed his eyes tight and began. Matter-of-fact at first.

"It's gonna sound trivial to some of you, but I don't give a shit anymore. I had an animal. I had her twenty-one years. A tabby cat that lived in my house. That fucking cat followed me everywhere. No matter what kind of mood I was in she was there. If I watched television she sat next to me on my chair. When I showered she was outside the curtain. When I slept she curled next to me. And when I talked on the phone or read the paper or ate breakfast she was there. Didn't matter what was happening with my wife or my kids or my brother. She was the first thing I saw in the morning and the last at night."

He paused and twisted his lip. Kept his eyes squeezed tight. "She was the first fucking thing that really loved me no matter what. And I swear I loved her, too. As much as I ever loved anyone. I loved that fucking tabby cat. She died, this time of year, four years ago. . . . Fucking cat. Since then, every now and then, I think I hear her mewing outside or when I'm almost asleep I think she's curled up next to me." And he smiled, his face twisted up, and laughed, at first just a sad chuckle. But then harder, and harder, until he was guffawing, and I smiled, and then laughed, and soon we were all laughing. He snorted, "Fucking cat."

Fourteen days before our wedding, and fifteen days before we moved our entire lives to California for my last chance at a cure, Terry phoned me late at night. I was asleep when she called. She'd just finished the three-to-twelve shift at the hospital and her car had a flat tire, she said. I threw on some clothing and drove to the parking garage where I found her struggling to loosen the lug nuts on her front left tire. We heard something coming from nearby, a high-pitched mewing sound. I told her to ignore it. Terry stood up and wandered toward the little voice.

She returned a few moments later carrying a kitten. "Look, it's adorable!" she cooed. I told her to put it down. Who knows where it belonged. It could have feline leukemia or worse. "Oh, just look at her, she's so cute!" Terry said, holding the cat up as evidence. I didn't want to look at it, knowing where this could lead. After all, we already had two cats at home.

Then Terry did one of the most manipulative things she's ever done to me. "Here," she said. "Hold it." And she handed me the cat. It fit into one hand and looked up at me. It had a small face with bright yellow eyes. It had six toes on each paw. I felt my resolve weaken. With one last Herculean effort I put the animal on the ground and was about to walk away when it rolled on its back and mewed playfully, showing a furry belly. It read me like a cheap paperback. Terry said, smiling, "We'll call her Hope." She lifted the kitten up and wrapped it in her shirt.

In California, as in the bone marrow transplant unit, my world grew small. I rarely left the apartment as the weeks crawled on. The cats lived there with us. Hope found every inch of the apartment fascinating. When I felt ill, which was much of the time, I'd watch and learn with her. She'd play with anything she found — paper, crumbs, shirts, blankets, window shades, and insects. Fully engaged in life.

But when I was the sickest, fighting the really hard side effects, Hope would sit beside me as still as a great oak on a calm day. In the bathroom, in the bedroom, in the little kitchen. If I was in anguish, I'd look up and she'd be sitting right next to me. Always. A great fucking cat.

Night of Fire

My body temperature has climbed past 106 degrees and the world is slowing. A young resident, in charge of my care, is at the end of my bed, talking in hushed tones to a nurse. His stethoscope is casually wrapped around his neck and he gesticulates while he speaks. From his gestures I think he is talking about treatment options. He is saying I could have this or that. The nurse nods in agreement and then bites her lip. He need not whisper. I know what he's saying. I know what's happening inside my body. I'm dying. I'm more certain of this than I've been of anything in my life. It's irrefutable and the terrible weight of my impending demise crushes every other fledgling thought from consciousness.

I am wrapped in a plastic blanket filled with a cold liquid. I am freezing from the inside out. To me, the hospital room at 70 degrees feels as if it's 30 below zero. My joints are stiff from the cold, my breathing is labored and fast. A moment ago I stopped shaking as my body climbed out of the rigor zone, from 103 past 104 and 105 and now, 106. With each ascending degree there was a host of new reality-altering symptoms. At 102 I felt my skin crawl. At 103 I couldn't stop myself from shaking. At 104 it was hard to draw breath. At 105 the world slowed. Now, at 106, I'm losing my ability to focus and understand.

The resident turns to me. He has mastered the art of efficient communication drilled into young physicians from the moment they get to medical school. Just the facts, look calm, look professional. Never mind that you are panicked and confused.

"The Tylenol hasn't seemed to do anything to reduce the fever, we're going to try some other ideas," he says.

I try to respond, but my mind is painfully slow. What is he saying? Tylenol? To save my life? It seems laughable and I smile at him. He furrows his brow in confusion. "Do you understand?"

Of course, I think to myself, but I'm not sure I do. I try to tell him that I understand. "Uhhh . . ."

The technical term for my condition is bacterial sepsis. A result of months of living with no immune function. The bacteria naturally living in my bowel have wormed their way into my bloodstream and I am poisoned and dying. When bacteria get into the bloodstream, they act like food coloring dropped in water. Quickly the entire body of liquid changes. In an effort to excise the bacteria from my system my body has heated itself. I have no other defenses. No natural killer cells to destroy offending invaders.

The resident starts a mental status exam by asking me simple questions. Mental status exams are designed to assess the cognitive functioning of patients. They're a quick and dirty assessment device that every clinical psychology graduate student and medical student learns and can eventually do in his or her sleep.

The resident leans toward me and asks me where I am. He has a mole on his cheek and it seems to float there. It looks familiar. It's a lighthouse on a foreign shore. I know I'm in the hospital, but then I'm not sure. I wonder for a moment. Am I at home? This room looks so familiar.

"Am I at home?" I ask him. The nurse at the end of the bed slowly shakes her head no and purses her lips.

"Wait a minute, I'm not at home. . . ." I mutter, but the words feel jumbled and come out only with great effort. I can see that he can't understand what I'm saying. And then the terrible realization strikes. I'm failing a mental status exam. I've given hundreds of these to patients and only those with significant neurological problems ever fail. But my mind and this room are falling away. I must be dying. My brain is stopping. Right now.

There was a tire commercial on when I had my first premonition that I was dying.

I was ten weeks into Stanford 5. Stanford 5 was the name assigned to the eight chemotherapeutic drugs put together into an experimental treatment regimen for advanced Hodgkin's disease. It was designed to be a heavy treatment for newly diagnosed patients.

The menu included the following: Adriamycin. (Heart toxic. It's a bright red liquid. The first time it was hung on my I.V. pole, an older patient leaned toward me and said, "Gettin' the 'red death,' huh? You hang in there, ya hear?" Before the days of Zofran, a terrific antinausea drug, Adriamycin resulted in two days of steady vomiting.) Bleomycin. (Rashes developed on my thighs.) Vinblastine. (Caused nerve damage.) VP-16. (My insides sloughed off.) Prednisone. (Puffy cheeks, nightmares, moodiness, depression.) Cyclophosphamide. Nitrogen mustard. Vincristine.

I got hit with at least two of these drugs each week. After the first week I was starting to feel better when they hit me the second time. The third hit felt too early, much too soon. I was still sick, flulike, from the second hit. My bone marrow had tired from the two full courses of chemo I'd already had, as well as the radiation and the bone marrow transplant. I knew before I started Stanford 5 that it might kill me, that it was designed for people who'd never had chemotherapy. But it was my last chance to be cured. Still, I thought of leaving. Unlike many patients who want to die fighting, I wanted to die at home, surrounded by the people who love me.

But I stayed. By the eighth week I'd been in the hospital twice with dangerous infections. I felt as if I'd aged seventy years. Earth's gravitational pull had been turned up. I couldn't walk up stairs or open doors. I took measured steps. I cursed people who bumped into me even slightly. *Don't they realize they could knock me down?* I was better when Terry was with me, but she'd found a job two hours away in Sacramento, where she worked three days a week. We needed the money so I learned to spend time alone.

Sometime after ten A.M., I notice the first spots flickering and dancing in front of my eyes. These are new. I am mildly entertained by them, as I was when I found the longitudinal hairline that ran down my leg from my thigh to my ankle. On the right side no hair grew. On the left side my leg was covered with as much hair as ever. My very own timberline.

A little while later I feel the telltale sign of a fever. Fire and ice running up and down my arms. I take my temperature. It's only one hundred. No big deal. I'm watching the news: Jerry Brown holds up a telephone number on a placard and asks people to send him money so he can go to Washington and save the planet. He wears a soft sweater and I feel he's someone I might want to have a beer with.

During the commercials that follow it occurs to me that something is terribly wrong. It's a conviction. A fact. I wonder if I should phone Terry, but I realize I have nothing substantial to say. I'd just interrupt her busy day at work. She'd whisper into the phone, "What's up?" and I'd say, "I think something horrible is happening," and she'd say, "What are your symptoms?" and I'd respond, "I have a mild fever and I think I'm dying," and she'd say, "What else aside from the fever?" and I would say, "Uh, nothing," and she'd say, "Dan, I love you, honey, but you have to let me get some work done," and I'd hang up and feel like an idiot. So I don't call. I watch a few more minutes of television and then decide to get the thermometer again. A hundred and one. Hah. Now we're getting somewhere. If it hits 102, I can call her and have something substantial to say.

I feel chilled. Sure sign of a fever. Dan Quayle is on now, sounding surprisingly articulate until someone asks him a question and he smirks dumbly and pauses too long before answering. I wonder if I can spot the poor bastard standing near him who's thinking, Dan, just say it the way we practiced. Oh shit. Oh shit. I search the faces behind Quayle, but they are all nodding and smiling.

I am dying. The thought creeps into my consciousness again, waving a blood-red flag. The phone rings, interrupting morbid ruminations. Thank God! I wheeze and pick myself up off the futon, shedding my friendly blankets. *Ring.* It feels cold out from under the blankets. Even colder than normal. Ice age again so soon? *Ring.* Whose idea was it to put the phone on this table so far away? "Hello?"

Ah, Terry. Savior. I tell her there is something wrong. I just don't feel right. She is supportive. She tells me to call a cab and go to the emergency room. I don't want to. I'm not sure I'm strong enough to make it down the stairs. But I'm also afraid to tell her the real reason I'm reluctant to go, that I'm sure I'll die on plastic seats in a rusting yellow car in the middle of a California freeway with some guy saying, "Hey, buddy, you okay? You don't look so hot. HEY BUDDY?" She sounds worried. She'll leave work now and it will take her a few hours to get here. I didn't mean to worry her so much, or did I?

I hang up and check the thermostat. It's far too cold to be seventy-five degrees. It feels as if it's fifty. Is this damned thing broken? Spots return and drift lazily across my field of vision. My teeth start to chatter. Shit. I feel tired, too tired. Rest sounds good. Maybe just a quick nap.

Gonna die today.

Can't think that way. I get up from the blankets and find my favorite sweater. It has a heavy cotton stitch, modeled after sailors' sweaters. I concentrate on getting each arm into it. I feel so frail. If this is what being very old feels like, I'd just as soon skip it and wait for the movie to come out.

Back in the living room, Paul Tsongas is being interviewed. A cancer survivor. He looks good, but I have the sneaking feeling he's hiding something. The way he puts so much effort into making eye contact and not blinking when he says, "My health is excellent." Has he relapsed? Now someone is talking about one of the Bush children who keeps getting into trouble.

By the time Terry gets home, I've dozed off. I wake up when she comes in. Her face is rosy and her chest heaves from being out of breath. She's in a business suit. She looks angelic. Sweet Teresa. Why is this happening to you? You don't deserve this. The cats seem to agree. They hop down from around me and purr as they rub her legs. She phones the oncology floor of the hospital, hoping that we can avoid the emergency room. We huddle together and she helps me out the door and down the forty-two steps to the waiting car. Inside the car I put the seat down and gather blankets around me. Every now and then I feel my teeth start to chatter and I stop them. Terry doesn't need to hear them while she's driving. When she's afraid she drives erratically.

This is probably just some sort of bug, some sort of virus that will be gone soon. This is the third week in a row I've been to the emergency room, and I haven't died yet; it's childish to feel so frightened this time. Have I become one of those nervous hypochondriacs who will haunt his doctors, forever complaining about some elusive twitch? The spots are no longer dancing across my vision. That's comforting. I must be getting better. Typical. I feel horrible at home and get to the hospital feeling fine. They'll think I just want attention.

Terry parks the car and runs around to open my door. "Chivalry is not dead!" I chirp, but the words vibrate and they sound too forced. She giggles for a moment as if I have said something hysterical and we walk in, huddled together, masquerading as a couple whose lives are idyllic.

In the emergency room they take my temperature. A hundred and three. Hah! I do have a right to be here! Vindication. They usher me to the oncology floor, where I will be admitted for the night. A resident wants to take my blood. I argue with him. My veins are tired, most are no longer visible and the ones I can see are blue lines as thin as hair. He insists and I give in. I should know better: Junior residents can't hit my veins; I need experienced older nurses with thick hands and attitudes. An eager medical student appears, no doubt charged with extracting a social history. He starts asking the usual questions. He's a gentle guy but I have no patience. I answer a few and then stare at him. "Read my chart. There's a great history and physical from January. Get what you need there, 'cause I'm not answering any more questions now." The resident huddling over my veinless appendages laughs at this. Terry stands by in her business suit looking exhausted and out of place. She approaches me from behind the medical student. "Honey, you're gonna stay the night, I'm gonna go back home and grab some comfortable clothing and a toothbrush. Back soon." And she's gone. The resident gives up after jabbing me a few times for good measure, and leaves, humiliated, to search for a nurse. Not sure what to do next, the medical student stands awkwardly like a boy waiting to ask for a dance. Eventually he turns and leaves too. I am alone.

Now I slacken my jaw and let my teeth resume their chattering. They generate a Morse code only they understand. My body begins to shake too. In medicine they call these rigors. I'm a human earthquake. Perhaps there is a human Richter scale to measure the violence of these jerks and twitches? If they could hook me up to a generator I could power this floor for a week. I giggle.

A nurse appears. She has the seasoned look of a veteran; hospital service pins cover her lapels. She eyes my blankets with skepticism. Uh-oh. First she finds veins. "It's great to work with pros," I compliment her. She is unswayed. She drops the bomb. "No more blankets," she says and pulls them gently from my bed, revealing my scrawny body.

I protest, "You're kidding, it's Arctic in here! I heard Iditarod racers mushing through a minute ago!" She leaves, taking my blankets with her. Smart woman. With the blankets gone the cold sets in. My bones are refrigerant pipes and I freeze from the inside out. I shake more violently and my teeth chatter accelerates. Terry should be back soon. The ceiling has small holes in random patterns.

The nurse is back with a thermometer. A hundred and four. It's climbing steadily. A fog is settling in my head like the thick vapors that descend after a New England snow melt. It takes a few seconds longer to hear words and register meaning. The nurse is saying something about "cold packs." How ridiculous, she's talking about beer at a time like this. She leaves, apparently to get the beer. Cold pack? Oh shit. She's talking about my bed. She's going to pack my bed with a cold sheet! A minute later she's back with a few other nurses. "Get out of bed," the mob insists. "Go away, you got my blankets, my wallet is over there," I plead. "OUT!" the alpha nurse roars. "Don't you have anything else to do? Isn't there a small child you could harass around here somewhere?" Arms grab me to help me out of bed and I struggle to keep my balance. One of the younger nurses lays a soft plastic sheet filled with a liquid on the bed. Another plugs something in. A machine begins to hum nearby. A few help me get back on the bed which is now as cold as my insides. As the sheet cools the fog clears. Now I'm pissed. "This is barbaric. This can't be necessary! You're going to give me pneumonia with this shit!" The alpha nurse has heard this sort of protest before.

Where's Terry?

The bed is freezing. The dots are back, writhing across my visual field.

The resident reappears and huddles with alpha nurse and the other nurses at the foot of my bed. They look frightened. There is no casual chatter mixed amongst the Latin medical phrases. They are somber and guarded. One bites her lower lip. Something is very wrong. Someone from outside the room cracks open the door and whispers in to them. Is that Terry's voice I hear? Are they keeping her from me? I've seen them do this on intensive care units, keeping a relative from a dying patient because the family member is in the way when things get dicey. I tell the alpha nurse to let me see my wife. She tells me she hasn't returned yet. I know she's lying. I heard Terry's voice, didn't I? I think I did. Poor Terry. If they're keeping her out of the room, she must know how grave my condition is. I wonder if I should rip the I.V. out of my arm and rush the door. Show her I'm okay. They tell me to relax, to calm down, everything is fine. But they look worried, similar to parents pacifying a child who knows too much.

Maybe they're telling the truth? If they are and Terry isn't here then I'm paranoid? I know that paranoids often cause the things they fear most. Professionals organize together to stop paranoid people from hurting themselves or others. But all the paranoid sees is a conspiracy. Is that why they're whispering? Am I paranoid?

They've agreed on something. The resident starts a mental status exam. Where I live and where I am. "Am I at home?" When the nurse shakes her head no, I feel the bed falling. I can hear the resident, but I can't communicate anymore. I don't care. I'm tired. My eyes are focusing on whatever they choose. Poor Teresa. What will she do now?

Someone is taking my temperature again. "Forty-one point five Celsius, a hundred and six point five," a clipped female voice says. She continues talking, asking a question I think, but I can't understand her anymore. There are many people around. I know the end is coming. I see myself intubated and on a ventilator. A purple tube is shoved deep into my throat. It delivers air to my lungs because my body will no longer do this on its own. They've paralyzed me with curare so that I won't yank the tube from my throat. Because I'm paralyzed I can't feel myself breathing. I wonder if I'm drowning, airless, in my own fluids. In this fantasy I feel a small hand on my forehead and hear my wife's voice. I don't want to die. If I cling to the rails of this bed, will death still take me? I hear my heart, pounding heavy and slow in my temples. There are urgent voices around me. I don't care about them. But there's someone else, too? There's a real hand on my forehead, isn't there? It's so gentle. So small. I want to curl into it. I want it to lift me away, up into the ether. It's a beacon and I turn my whole being toward it. Fingertips move slowly along my brow. Stopping here, visiting there. They're in no rush. Maybe I'll just stay awake a few moments longer. "It's all okay," the hand tells me. "You've been so strong. You can rest now."

Warmth. The sound of Terry's familiar breathing nearby. My chest and back are soaked. There's bright light everywhere. I'm under a sheet but don't need it. I squint my eyes toward a voice. Terry is smiling at me.

"Hey, sweetie," she says. "You feel up for some breakfast?"

Hurricane Andrew's Pupils

I looked down into the green blanket. Treetops and swamp gave way to two-lane roads and tin roofs. The pilot said we were getting closer. Buckle up. The landscape changed abruptly. Suddenly there were downed trees zigzagging like toothpicks across the road. There were overturned trucks and exposed dollhouse walls and mud and shingles. There were crumpled steel power trestles that resembled squatting old men. They reminded me of brown-faced Italians hunched over dice in the alley near my boyhood home in Newark.

The prop plane started its descent. There were nine of us on board including the pilot. Six clinical psychology faculty, a psychology intern, and me, the lone graduate student. It was eleven months before Terry and I would leave for California, and three days after Hurricane Andrew struck. I'd become interested in the best ways to help people through crises. I'd done relief work after the Gainesville student murders and a faculty member had asked me to join our departmental crisis team a few days after the hurricane.

As we descended I tied a shoelace and wondered about finding my possessions strewn across my front lawn. How I'd feel if I needed a neighbor to help me pull out of the mud and insulation the touch lamp I found at the flea market, my Vassar Ultimate Frisbee T-shirt, or a birthday card scrawled in my father's hand.

The plane set down, stopped, and the loud buzzing engine shut off. The pilot wrestled with the door for a few moments and then we gathered our bags and stepped into a wall of South Florida humidity. I squinted into a dark blue, cloudless sky. At the end of the runway planes were scattered about like children's toys. One leaned through the steel door of a hangar as if it had punched its wing through, looking for something inside. Another was upside down. When we got closer I could see that it was colored a dull silver and was speckled with chips of white paint. The pilot pointed at it. "The wind did that, took paint off everything, better than a sandblaster, huh?"

Outside the small airport we were welcomed by the coordinator of the university's agricultural program in Homestead. He was wearing jogging shorts and a T-shirt. I suspected it wasn't his normal work clothing. He thanked us profusely. He had a heavy Southern accent. Alabama maybe.

"Hope your flight was uneventful," he told us. "Y'all know we appreciate your making the long trip down from Gainesville. Everyone'll be waiting for ya. As I told y'all on the phone, we're hoping you folks can lend us some guidance. Some of our people have had the hardest four days of their lives."

We rode with the coordinator in a large van to the agriculture center. He took us through the last four days, starting with the weather advisories. When Hurricane Andrew struck Homestead, the wind speeds were higher than 175 miles per hour. I thought of Ray Romero, the pitcher on our high-school baseball team who could throw eighty-five miles an hour. It seemed that the instant the ball left his hand it was popping into the catcher's mitt. "It was like a big tornado," the coordinator said.

As we drove toward the agriculture center, the randomness became obvious. Andrew had wrapped a steel girder around a tree but left an old wooden mailbox untouched. It had overturned a long recreational vehicle, but the trailer next door hadn't budged from the bricks on which it rested.

The army was arriving. Jeeps sat at a few of the intersections and troops scurried about. Young men in full battle fatigues directed us to wait and then proceed. Sitting at one of the intersections I noticed that most houses had spray-painted street names and house numbers in large block letters across them. Some had messages to family members: *Grandma is fine* or *We R OK, Thank Jesus.* Others were warnings: *WILL SHOOT LOOTERS AGAIN.* I craned my neck taking it all in.

The clinical director discussed our plan. Though we'd talked about it on the plane, her reviewing it in the midst of the chaos outside the vehicle was comforting. It reminded me of our purpose. The goal of crisis debriefing is to allow individuals who have experienced a traumatic event to have their perspective validated and, where possible, normalize their emotional response. We've learned since Vietnam that when people are exposed to trauma and no one says, "That was a terrible thing you survived," post-traumatic stress is compounded. I've always thought of crisis debriefing as resetting someone's emotional compass, like pointing a lost hiker north. We do this by giving folks a chance to tell their stories, and letting them know that it's normal during a crisis to feel completely overwhelmed. To be numb or rage or cry or withdraw or feel crazy. After trauma we all need to know that what we went through was beyond the realm of normal experience and that it's okay to feel nothing or everything.

We arrived at the agriculture center. It was a set of modest, one-story buildings surrounded by cultivated land; there were offices, garages, and sheds scattered across a few acres. The center was the command post for an ambitious research program designed to assist agricultural efforts in the state of Florida. The center tested innovations in growing common crops and then shared the successful methods with farmers across the state. The center employed many Homestead residents who worked jobs like those on any large farm. They planted, harvested, and kept the place going.

The clinical director approached me and said she and I would work with a group of older black farmhands. We called out names and greeted one another. To a man, they were broad-shouldered and strong, with an average age of about forty. Together we found a corner of a garage and sat in a circle. We parked ourselves on whatever we could find—seed bags, grain boxes—and a few just sat between oil stains on the concrete floor. The aluminum roof overhead was scarred and light streamed through, producing a hole of light in the middle of the circle.

We decided that each man would tell his story, uninterrupted, until everyone had spoken. There was some jostling and silence, but eventually one of the men said he would go first.

He spoke simply, with no drama or visible emotion. He'd held the door to his bathroom shut while his home disappeared around him, his wife and child wrapped together in the tub. When he was done there was quiet nodding all around. No one coughed, or changed positions, and I wondered if this was what church felt like during a powerful sermon.

The second man described the wind. He leaned forward, slow tears descending down the craggy landscape of his cheeks, and spoke slowly and softly with a Cuban accent. "It was a train. God's train. It was so loud, we cover our ears and close our eyes." For a moment I imagined huddling with Terry under our coffee table as a silver engine streaked through our Gainesville apartment, ripping our lives away.

The third man was older. He had come outside during the eye of the storm, a period of brief calm, and realized his neighborhood was fine. He laughed at the silliness of his brother-in-law who lived next door and had covered his kitchen window with a thin piece of plywood.

"I grew up in North Carolina. I been through Hazel in '54, Dianne in '55, and Agnes in '72," he chuckled. "Ain't no piece of mill plywood ever done no good." Then the eye moved on and the storm came back. When he fought through the debris in his living room to look out his front door he found the nose of his pickup truck emerging from his brother-in-law's window next door.

"Told him plywood ain't gonna do no good." Everyone laughed.

The fourth man told his story, and the fifth, sixth, and seventh, until there was one man left. In his mid-thirties I guessed, he was the biggest man of the group. He was well over six feet four, with broad shoulders. His skin was dark ebony, interrupted only by a jagged scar from his mouth to near his left ear. His eyes were red rimmed and tired and his thick lips were chapped. He tilted his head, looking up into the sky through the crack in the roof and told his story in a steady rhythmic baritone.

His house was spared, but like everyone else, his electricity had been lost. His wife was pregnant and the loss of air conditioning was taking a toll. They'd started having arguments. A few days after Andrew's exit, a power company crew from South Carolina arrived in his neighborhood. They'd driven three trucks down in twelve hours nonstop. They started rewiring Homestead. The rumble of their trucks could be heard in his neighborhood in the early hours of the morning. He heard the voices outside. Neighbors had told him they were working morning and night, with only brief rests, all of them volunteers.

He stopped for a moment and then looked up. "I'm not a generous man," he said. "I don't volunteer extra hours, I don't cover other people's shifts, I don't work if we don't need the money," and his gaze found everyone.

When his air conditioner kicked back to life and his lights flickered on, the power company electric truck was just down his street. He thought about what they'd done, realized he would probably not have done the same, and wanted to thank them for their generosity. He headed out the door and down the road. About half a mile away he found the workers. There were men up in a lift, others talking on radios, and one pointing to a clipboard and shouting up directions. He was only fifty feet or so away when he realized all of them were white.

He'd rehearsed a few phrases, a simple thank-you. When he arrived at the truck, the men stopped working and looked at him. Suddenly he couldn't speak. His thank-you wouldn't come. He stood for a long time saying nothing. The strangers on the truck squinted at him and he wondered if they were fearful or angry — whites often responded to him like that, a big black man in stained work clothes. His words were frozen and he worried, until one of the men put a hand on his shoulder and said, "It's all right, man, you're welcome," and he realized that despite the absence of words, his thank-you had arrived in his eyes, his shoulders, and his pursed lips.

When we lived outside of Palo Alto, Terry worked as a consultant, three days a week, in Sacramento. She drove two hours, each way, to get there. Her work brought in money we desperately needed. The money from our wedding ran out quickly. My parents helped as much as they could and Vassar alumni helped, too. All were generous, but the money was gone after eight weeks. When Terry went to Sacramento I was alone in the apartment.

I knew on some primal level that I'd lose what I didn't use. That I had to leave the apartment, gain back some semblance of independence. Leaving the apartment required assessing the weather, dressing correctly, and eating something for energy. But more than planning, it required bravery, the kind of bravery that allowed boys to charge from their foxholes across a bright open field. In my case, I feared I lacked the energy and strength to make it back to the apartment.

Eventually I realized I never felt that fear when Terry was around. When we went walking, I felt strong, confident, unbeatable. She was a buoy I clung to in a treacherous sea.

Terry had been a bone marrow transplant nurse for eleven years. The nurses who worked for her used to say she always knew when death was coming for a patient, usually long before anyone else. Every so often I saw my death in her emotions, her slow, subtle pulling away. Then she'd tumble back, as if she were the tides and I her beach.

I remember watching her on our small balcony, her hands on the banister, her face looking out. Her eyes so weary. And then an almost imperceptible gesture, a movement of her hand, a tired slow drift through the air that ended with her hand touching her neck. She was too exhausted to hold me up much longer.

And all I felt was gratefulness, appreciation for everything she'd given and endured with me — marrying me despite knowing this could be coming, moving across the country to a desolate apartment, walking with me every night. Standing outside the bathroom door. Petting my head while I tried to find sleep.

I didn't thank her then. I wanted to but I couldn't yet. I couldn't put words on what I felt and I didn't have the energy to reach out. I knew I should but I didn't. Watching her outside on that balcony, I couldn't help but admire the courage of the big man from Homestead who stood wordless on the side of the road, his shoulders bobbing in the Florida heat, his eyes filled with salt and gratitude.

Gallium Oracle

My mother's relatives responded in different ways to the Holocaust. Nana's sister sought solace in God; her descendants, my cousins, aunts and uncles, are conservative Jews. Nana, in contrast, believed that a God could not exist and allow the systematic eradication of her family.

I didn't attend Hebrew school. Wasn't Bar Mitzvahed. Instead I was taught to put faith in science and action. My politics were born of a central belief: My mother's family and others allowed the Nazis to rise to power with too little opposition. The next time we would be active instead of passive. Fight first and pray later. Passive resistance was dangerously inadequate when matched against an evil and persuasive tyrant such as Hitler.

My father's side was comprised of practical immigrants. The ways of the old country were quickly abandoned in favor of bookkeeping and managing stores. My grandfather was facile with numbers and found work as an accountant. My grandmother was a writer and worked as a teacher.

Of things Jewish in both families, only stories and recipes were passed down. The stories, like how Uncle Julius survived in Dachau and Buchenwald by remembering his wife, or how cousins skied the Alps to escape the Nazis. And food—how to make kugel, challah, gefilte fish.

I had no formal spiritual training. No guiding laws about faith. And no expectation that life should be easy or end well. Instead of religious teaching I learned from the scientific and political books lining the walls of my childhood home. Physics. Chemistry. Astronomy. Mathematics . . . Zionism. Communism. Socialism. Fascism. When in doubt, look to yourself or science for guidance. Superstition, astrology, prayer, and even hope had no place on those bookshelves.

Hodgkin's tumors love gallium, a radioactive isotope. They drink it up. Then they're easy to scan. By January of 1992 I'd been gallium-scanned five times, roughly once a year for five years. Each time the tumor in my chest had lit up like a warning flare.

And each time my oncologist tried to explain it. He'd fumble around with some way to keep my spirits up without misleading me. Turning off the light box, he'd mumble, "Well it doesn't nec- essarily mean that it's growing or not growing. It's probably grow- ing, but nodular sclerosing tumors leave behind scar tissue, maybe the scar tissue absorbed some of the . . ." But we both knew that if the tumor was dead, it wouldn't light up. Otherwise there wouldn't be any point to the scan.

I grew accustomed to bad news or, at best, ambiguous news from scans and biopsies. I tried to make them as routine as hospi- tal parking problems, insurance claim forms, or strange side effects. I learned to tune them out, to base my impressions of my progress more on how I felt than on the pessimistic messengers of modern science. If you feel like you're dying, look like you're dying, and act like you're dying, you're probably dying. If not, you're probably living. Simple. As Nana might have said with a shrug. But at night the terror of my gradual demise and the steady flow of bad news was inescapable.

In January, three weeks after my night of fire, I again accepted that my death was inevitable. My body was deteriorating before me. I'd lost forty pounds. I could no longer open doors or climb stairs without help. I moved more slowly, awkwardly. I slept more. Ate less.

I started saying good-bye to things. For me, the dying process was about letting go of memories and the emotions each evoked while my body slowly stopped. Facing death felt like a skill I couldn't quite master. I tried saying these good-byes without slipping into sentimental gushiness, but it was challenging. The smallest memory, of a red umbrella on a beach in the morning summer sun, could elicit overwhelming emotion. The red umbrella reminded me of vacationing with my parents in South Jersey, and then I'd be thinking of that memory, imagining myself playing with David for hours in the sand and the horrifying idea of saying good-bye to him.

Eventually I started keeping a list, akin to those I might take to the supermarket. Every time I had a memory, an annoying inner voice interrupted with, *Well, this could be the last time you think about that, maybe it should go on the list,* and I'd have to scribble it down before I could allow myself to think about something else. I wrote while standing in a cashier line, and again on a walk, and while watching a movie. I might jot down: *Dry wooden floating docks at Camp Woodstock where I learned to canoe, tangled frizzy ends of my first girlfriend's brunette hair.* A few days later, *Snowballs packed just right, like when David and I had the snowball fight with Peter across the street. My leather boots wet from the rains when I camped alone in Maine.* The list grew and grew; it was unmanageable in no time.

Terry's impossibly clean bird cages. The pock-riddled stop sign at the end of my street when I was little. Lox bits my father brought home from the bakery on Sunday mornings. The smoky smell of my flannel shirts after skiing with Roland and his brothers in Vermont. Buttered popcorn. The easy melodies of James Taylor and Vivaldi when I was getting chemotherapy. Raw untempered fucking and wet sweaty backs. Subway trains with flickering lights when my father took me into New York City when I was just old enough to walk. Old men with brown paper bags who lingered on the street corner near my childhood home in Newark. Spider lightning across the sky when I left a movie theater holding my grandfather's coat. My brother's eyes. My mother's hands.

Radiology suites are different from most other parts of a hospital. Unlike the outpatient oncology floors and the inpatient units, which are designed to have the look and feel of patient areas, the radiology suites are where laboratory and patient care meet. Like caged beasts, huge machines fill their own rooms. Anterooms are stuffed with computers and monitors. Like futuristic pilots, attendants bathed in blue light sit with headphones at computer screens. On my way to the scan room I passed closets marked with the same radiation symbols seen at nuclear power stations, and workers wearing lab coats over shorts and sneakers.

An attendant checked my name. I asked, "How 'bout a gin fizz? Hmmm, no, the gin's no good here. How 'bout a black-and-tan? No, er . . . I've got it! Do you have something nuclear?" The attendant stared blankly at me. He pulled the needle from a lead case and injected me. I felt a familiar warmth. The gallium coated my insides with a neon glow.

After a two-hour wait I walked slowly back into the gallium scan room. The technician, a man with sad eyes and a gray pony-tail, directed me to the scanning table where I would lie prone and motionless for twenty minutes or so. He wore a lab coat with patches sewn on from other countries. Guatemala, Nigeria, Tibet. It was comforting. Traveling to so many places must have taken many years. If he'd worked here the entire time he was a gallium scan veteran. *And he's probably a dependable man*, I thought. Travelers can't afford to be mistake prone or unorganized.

I was too weak to climb onto the table by myself. I stood in front of it, motionless for a moment and he came up behind me.

"Uh, sorry, I could use a hand." My head turned downward. He lifted me up and onto the table. Firm hands. Sure. A backpacker?

"Thanks," I muttered, embarrassed by my weakness.

"It's no problem," he assured me. Genuine.

He disappeared behind a door and I was alone for a moment. I could read the GE symbol on the scanner. A strange place to advertise, I thought. There was nothing on the ceiling. A true patient-centered scanning room would have a collage on the ceiling. Something engaging to look at, maybe even an entire story in pictures. A monitor hummed awake near my feet. I hadn't noticed it before. I'd be able to watch the results with him. To see my tumor when it lit up. He was close to me again. He put a hand on me and said softly, "Don't move, I'll get you out of here quick, I promise." And he retreated out of view. I kept my eyes on the monitor.

I could hear beeps from across the room—was he punching numbers into a computer? The scanner jerked to life. It slowly moved over me. Then he stepped to the monitor. I waited. He drank from a small cup using both hands while the heavy machine moved over and around me. Soup? Hmmm. I noticed my own hunger. Good to be hungry. Eating is part of life. Need to eat more. I clicked my teeth to a Beatles song in my head. "You say you want a revolution . . . yeah ah, you know . . ." What should I have for breakfast?

"Can you see this?" he asked me.

"Yeah," I said. The scan was almost over. He was pointing to the monitor. My upper torso was displayed in outline and the gallium was gathering in various organs, highlighting them. Oh good, I thought. He knows something. Some veteran technicians pretend they don't know what they're looking at. "You need to talk to your doctor about that," they'd deadpan. I often coaxed them to show me the scans. I'd even bully them.

"Look, it's my body, not the doctor's, I have a right to see them. Come on, I won't tell anyone I saw them. . . ."

I'd hold them up to the light or put them on the nearest display board. With X rays I'd press my hands up to the scan and count the width of the mother tumor in fingers.

"It's five fingers wide when the chest is two hands across," I might announce. During the first round of chemo I scribbled the information down and studied it later. After the relapses I stopped watching as closely.

I steadied myself for the results. The tumor would light up next. It would stare back at me the same size as always, the unflinching fuck. *But who cares what this scan says, right? Doesn't mean you're dying. It's all okay. You're not dead until you're dead.*

Here we go. The technician pointed. "Here's your rib cage, here's your spleen—they let you keep your spleen, huh?" he asked. Impressive. Most techs don't know this much about Hodgkin's disease.

"Yeah," I was saying when I saw it. I steeled myself with clinical skepticism. *Doesn't necessarily mean anything,* I thought. *There's still a long way to go yet.* But the realization enveloped me. I felt an electric pulse in my temples and my throat closing. Tears welled up in my face and I tried to breathe.

"Here's your liver. . . ." he said. He was moving his hands up to my lungs, but his voice faded. My eyes squeezed shut. He was up to my neck now, pointing and talking softly. Then he was done. No more anatomy. And the tears dropped and I held my breath.

He stopped. Looked curiously at me. "Looks clean. Where was your tumor supposed to be?" I couldn't answer. Like a man emerging from years of solitary confinement who turns his face upward and squints toward the sun. I was basking in hope's reward for the first time.

Dictated Chart Note

4/92

The patient was treated at Stanford University with Stanford V, a MOPP/ABVD hybrid chemotherapy protocol. (This aggressive regimen was made possible by the advent of hematopoetic growth factors to prevent prolonged myelosuppression.)

The patient suffered a number of complications, not surprising given his history of heavy treatment. He developed gram negative bacteremia twice. The latter episode was severe and included septic shock, hypotension, cognitive deterioration, and reduced O_2 saturation. After recovering from bacteremia the patient received his final cycle of chemotherapy without complications. Following completion of chemotherapy the patient received an additional 2600cGy of mantle radiation therapy. His total mantle radiation dose has now reached its maximum at 5000cGy. During his course of radiation the patient developed a severe case of varicella zoster infection involving a thoracic dermatome. The patient was treated with high dose acyclovir and experienced a full recovery.

It should be noted that this represents treatment for the second relapse in this patient. While he received aggressive high dose therapy here there is only a remote chance of long term, disease-free survival. The patient will return home for follow-up.

JOSHUA SOKOL, M.D.
Stanford Medical Center

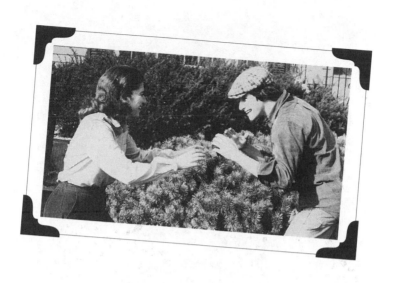

Part Six

The Years Since

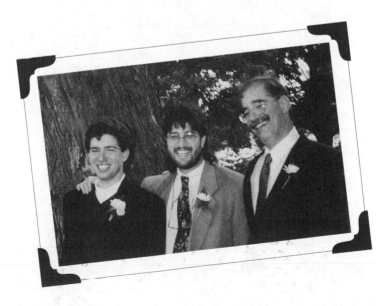

Slowball

Pat Morse is teaching me to ride. Pat is New England common sense. Grounded. Seasoned. And as I sit atop her thoroughbred, she's my guru. I've just begun my internship year in clinical psychology at McLean Hospital, a psychiatric teaching hospital affiliated with Harvard. I've completed my course work at the University of Florida and my internship is the last hurdle before I'll be awarded my Ph.D.

Already, despite being here for only two months, I am the primary caregiver, therapist, and dad for a broad collection of patients. Most of my patients are not sick enough to be in locked wards but are too mentally ill to live outside of the hospital. There's a professional alcoholic in for his ninety-first detox, a woman who cuts herself whenever she feels anxious, and a boy who lives at the extreme poles of depression and mania.

We're finding our way together. When I'm not running to meetings or answering phones I'm with my patients, sorting through today's insults and yesterday's haunting memories. Locked closets are opened, old rages are relived, and dreams that soar and crash are explored. But each haunting memory reminds me of my own. When the dissociative patient leans forward and whispers about the sound of broken glass in her childhood room, I think of the beeping machines on the bone marrow transplant unit. When the alcoholic tells me he can't shake the smell of bourbon, he awakens to it in the middle of the night, I remember the smell of antiseptic and unwashed bodies, my own bolt into wakefulness at three A.M. Sometimes the memories feel too real, like they've just happened, and I have to claw my way back so I can be present, validating, all there for these patients who sense every distraction, every nip of neglect. I'm often scared that I'm not present enough, that my memories eclipse my ability to put myself in my patients' shoes, that the balance is weighted too heavily with my own hauntings. Once, when Bill Pollack, a supervisor, and I reviewed a tape of my session, he pointed out that I hadn't been listening. "Where were you?" he asked. He didn't expect me to answer. But we both knew.

At night, after twelve-hour days, I make the forty-minute drive west into the country where Terry and I have rented a farmhouse from Pat and Bill Morse, who keep their horses in the barn behind us.

On this particular night, eight o'clock but the sun is still up, I sit atop Snowball, who never won a race but was fast enough to run and placed a few times at the track. Pat affectionately calls her Slowball, but I don't feel that Snowball and I are friendly enough yet for me to tease her this way.

Now Pat holds a red line that drifts upward toward the horse's bridle.

"Close your eyes and let the horse walk under you. She's not going anywhere," Pat tells me. My eyes closed, we walk in a small circle, in a *bubump, bubump* rhythm around a small circle as the summer evening air cools. Yesterday the horse threw me. I rolled in the dirt for a moment and saw slow hoofs moving away from me.

"I'll have to ask you to get back on now," Pat had said quietly, and so I did.

Bubump,

    bubump,

        bubump.

Pat's voice is confident. "Don't worry, you'll find your balance. . . ."

Finding Fault

The Dana Farber Cancer Institute's Jimmy Fund clinic is the nicest clinic I've ever seen for children. It's fed by New England's favorite charity, the Jimmy Fund. With one bicycle race alone they get more than nine million dollars every year. And they deserve it. They work miracles there. When you step off the elevators on the fourth floor, you see smiling cartoon characters painted on the walls. In the waiting room there are fish tanks and video games, tables with Popsicle sticks and glitter. The first time I saw the unit, I knew I wanted to work there.

After my internship at McLean I applied for an endowed fellowship in Medical Crisis Counseling based at an institute at Harvard Medical School. It was run by Gerry Koocher, one of the most respected psychologists I knew of, a man who had pioneered the psychological treatment of children with cancer. It was an honor and easily the most rewarding educational experience I'd had. Gerry allowed the fellows in his program to find placements in any of the Harvard teaching hospitals. One of the rotations was at the Dana Farber pediatric clinic.

Jeremiah, the first boy I was assigned, was eight. His older brother was dying of high-risk acute lymphoblastic leukemia. Jeremiah was referred when his teachers complained that he'd stopped participating at school. His mother told me he'd withdrawn into himself, had stopped playing with other kids and avoided his older brother.

I met Jeremiah, brought him back from the waiting room into my office, and we started. Therapy with preadolescents is usually best approached through play. In the world of play children can express themselves and plant clues to lead the adult to the heart of the matter. But Jeremiah would not play with me. I tried my best stuff first, Legos. I'd met very few eight-year-olds who could resist building a Lego car with rack-and-pinion steering and shock absorbers. He left the pieces sitting in the box. Then I tried puppets and board games, Nerf balls and Crayolas. He wouldn't respond. He sat, spinning in his chair, while I challenged him to throw the Nerf ball into my trash can, or draw his favorite thing, or whip me at checkers. For four sessions we did the same thing. He'd come back to my office and I'd offer something we could do and he'd sit, silent, spinning his chair.

Finally, during the fifth session, I caught a break. He saw two plastic dinosaurs on my desk and asked if we could play with those. "Absolutely!" I said. I told him the two dinosaurs were brothers and handed them to him. He surveyed them quietly. They were both tyrannosaurus models, complete with scales, big tails, and ferocious little hands. "This is the older one," he told me, holding one of them up and nodding his head.

Ten minutes later we were sprawled across the carpet in my office when Jeremiah banged one little plastic figure into the other. "Try HARDER!!" he yelled, his voice scratchy and violent. "IF YOU'D TRY HARDER AND BE NICER, THIS WOULDN'T BE HAPPENING!" And his tears dropped onto the carpet.

The idea that our thoughts can have an impact on our diseases is exciting. Research does indicate that banging our fists on the steering wheel during a traffic jam is related to the slow closing of the highway of vessels around our hearts, and tenderness and love can soothe our gastrointestinal tracts, nurturing an irritable bowel back to health.

The popular culture claims that with emotional will we can improve everything, even feel our way to health and wealth. Like the advertisements in newspapers from the 1880s offering Grandma's heal-everything elixir, these days our minds may offer the great panacea.

There is impressive evidence that the mind does impact our health. Asthmatics and arthritics who write about traumatic events often enjoy symptom relief, group therapy might prolong life in metastatic breast cancer patients, and sick mice can be conditioned to respond to saccharine as if it were chemotherapy. I've seen guided imagery turn a breach baby, so it could enter the world head first, and I've seen evidence from exercise stress tests and MUGA scans that folks with heart disease who learn to live without anger have happier and healthier hearts. But as exciting as these findings are, it's also true that the mind's power over biology has important limits. Placebos don't work 100 percent of the time, and even saints can die of cancer.

People's notions and speculations about why I got cancer were usually comforting, just not to me. "Maybe you were exposed to too much stress," one friend wondered. "I read some studies that said that you probably repressed your anger," a colleague speculated. "I've heard that people who don't deal with conflict in their families are more prone to . . ." another patient told me. And the most common, "I read a popular book by a doctor who said that when you aren't hopeful enough about life . . ."

These comments, from loving folk, left me with guilt. What had I done wrong? How had I damned my cells to such misery and put myself and my family members through such hell? Perhaps I hadn't thought positively enough? Friends and family had always admired my tenacity, but could it be that beneath the surface I was racked with self-doubt? Maybe I didn't express my anger? My mother would disagree; our yelling matches over curfews and chores were frequently short but impressive. Maybe life was too stressful? Down the street Clarissa's mom had tried to kill herself a few times and Clarissa was fine. Ned's dad, in the house behind ours, drank too much — that had to be worse. Maybe I was just weak?

I wasn't alone. Many of the patients with cancer I worked with were flooded with unhelpful speculations by their friends and family. There was the young man who was told by a friend that his cancer took one of his limbs because he'd returned to law school. Or the young woman who learned that cancer had visited her life because she hadn't stood up to her father. Or the old woman who whispered that she should have never divorced her abusive husband, God was paying her back for violating his commandments.

Gesturing to the plastic Tyrannosaurus rex in my hand, I told Jeremiah, "It's not about trying harder. I'm sure he's trying as hard as he can." Jeremiah looked at me curiously, wiping the salt fury from his face with his sleeve. He didn't seem to understand. "IT'S NOT HIS FAULT HE GOT CANCER," I insisted, too forcefully, jerking the plastic dinosaur in the air for emphasis. Jeremiah looked from me to the dinosaur, surprised by my vehemence. I was surprised, too. I looked from the little plastic figure to Jeremiah, and wondered who I was really talking about.

Hunter

I'm sitting on the Green Line T, the train I always take into work, and we are stopped outside of Newton. I don't know why the train has stopped. I've just awoken from a daydream, finding my hand pressed into my throat. Since I've started working around people with cancer again, it's a familiar place to find my hand.

I know every millimeter of my supraclavicular region, the landscape between my collarbones and chin. I often discover my hands doing their ritualized dance on my neck as if the appendages had their own consciousness. It's been three years since I was last treated, but the hand dance continues. Scanning for the disease. The great hunter looking for the beast.

And I'm a good hunter. Better than most oncologists.

The key is pressure. Hodgkin's nodes will reveal themselves, but only when we force ourselves into their homes. I press uncomfortably hard. I have a trace memory of the tumors that lived here. Smooth, dense, and fixed, as if they belonged there.

Now four fingers move, one at a time, like a centipede, slow. Meticulous. First my right hand inside my left collarbone. Then my left hand inside the right collarbone. Then both hands together up my neck and under my chin. Then down to the groin, starting at hipbones and traveling south. Tumor hunting is rhythmic and determined, like old men on the beach slowly swinging their metal detectors.

MFB: Measure for Box

The University of Miami's Department of Surgery is located in one of the busiest tertiary care hospitals in the country. Jackson Memorial Hospital has more than fifteen hundred beds, nine thousand parking spots, a few helicopter landing pads, sixty acres of buildings, and forty-eight different comprehensive clinical services.

My tour guide, a business manager in the Department of Surgery, listed the hospital's impressive credentials as we walked down a long hallway to my next interview. I'd found the job listing in the back of an academic magazine. The fellowship at Harvard was coming to an end and I needed to find work. Terry and I were both ready to leave Boston. Harvard was a great place to train, but jobs were scarce and Boston was very expensive. Terry generously offered to move wherever I could find an academic job. At Miami they were advertising for an educator, someone who could come into the Department of Surgery and help the young surgeons learn, both the scientific and human sides of medicine. I thought it sounded interesting and applied. I didn't tell my possible employers about my illness history. I was healthy and it wasn't relevant.

I interviewed with many of the faculty and one current resident. The resident was young and athletic looking. He had pale pink skin and small red blotches on his face, the product of spending too much time indoors under stress, I thought. He wore an aqua scrub top and his arms were muscular. When we shook hands I could feel his strength; he hadn't learned not to shake hands hard, like the older surgeons I met. His face was thin and shaped like a wolf's. After we spoke for a while, covering my plans for how I'd assist his department, he apologized for not knowing more about me and asked if I was a psychologist. I told him I was. He squirmed for a moment in his chair, like a boy at a fancy restaurant intimidated by too much cutlery.

"What's up?" I asked.

"I haven't talked to anyone about this, but it's something that happened the first night of my second year and it surprised me," he said, looking at me. "I guess I just wonder what you'd think about it. . . ." I nodded. There was an awkward pause and then he continued, "Well, I'd just finished my internship, my first year here. I thought my second year was going to be a breeze com-

pared to the internship—they worked us like dogs, I did hundred-
hour weeks the whole year. Anyway, that first night of my second
year I was on in the emergency room. The older residents told me
there'd be a lot of frequent flyers and gomers, so I didn't think it
would be a big deal." His descriptions of his patients caught me,
the way fabric sticks on a rosebush. I translated. *Frequent flyer*: a
patient who uses the emergency room for primary care, too poor
or too unorganized to get conventional primary care. *Gomer*:
elderly person with many chronic problems. As he spoke, I imagined real people sitting on plastic chairs in the emergency room,
faces pale, hands rubbing together. And I remembered shivering
on those chairs myself, waiting and waiting for someone to come.
I felt impatience and heat rising in my chest. *Who does he think
he is?*

He continued, "I was the first guy in my class to get 'brick
duty'—we get these walkie-talkies, they look like bricks, that pick
up the emergency crews all over Miami. If they want to bring
someone to Jackson Memorial, we coordinate the surgical part,
you know, tell them what to do in the cars. Like if they get some
MFB or a SHPOS who's high on crack and crashed a car, then we
talk 'em through it." I listened. Translated. *MFB, Measure for
Box*, as in measure the body for a coffin. *SHPOS*? I'd heard the
word before. What did it mean? I searched the memory banks.
Then it clicked. An acronym. *Sub Human Piece of Shit.* The heat
in my chest became a burn. *I can't listen to this anymore. . . .* I
started to stand up but he continued, oblivious to my movement,
"So the night was going okay, the emergency room was basically a
rock garden, there were a couple of demented gomers with bad
squash rot, and some frequent flyers. I was doin' okay and then the
bricks went off." He stopped for a moment. Cleared his throat and
pinched the bridge of his nose and kept his hand over his eyes for
a moment. "A paramedic called me from a helicopter. He told me
this kid, like fifteen years old, was run over by a train and had lost

his legs. They were air-vacing him in." His voice went soft and he stared into the table. Absently ran a finger across his lip. I slowly dropped back into my seat.

He continued, each word trickling out softly, "I didn't know what I was supposed to tell him, you know. A nurse was standing near me when the bricks went off. She listened to the paramedic and told me exactly what I should say, about saving the legs and stopping the bleeding and hanging an I.V., so I did. I repeated everything she told me, word for word. Then, twenty minutes later, the 'copter landed at Ryder. Me and two nurses met it and took the kid into the operating room. The kid was a chew-toy— there was blood everywhere, on the pilots and the baseboard, I mean everywhere. I'd never seen so much blood. When we got him into the O.R., one of the senior residents screamed at me 'cause I didn't have gloves on. I'd totally spaced.

"Anyway, so later, around four A.M., when the kid is still in the O.R. circling the drain, like a real MFB, and I'm back in the emergency room sleeping, the kid's parents show up. A nurse woke me up and told me I had to tell 'em what happened to their son— about him losing his legs and everything. She said it like I'd just killed her dog, real pissy like, so I marched over and told 'em their son had been hit by a train, had lost his legs, and was still in the operating room. Just like that. Totally matter-of-fact."

As if he were deflating, he sagged over the table until his forehead touched it. For a moment he didn't say anything and I could see a foggy pool of breath beneath his mouth on the table. As he sat there quietly, I imagined him standing in front of two parents, them pleading with their eyes while he barked out horrible facts. I wondered if his belly was tight when he told them or if his legs shook. "No one ever told me what to do." He spoke down into the table, his voice uneven. "They still haven't told us what to do." And he looked up at me as wide swaths of watery humiliation streaked across his cheeks.

During my training to become a health psychologist I worked in
five hospitals. Some of the best in the country. Four hospitals affiliated with Harvard Medical School and Shands at the University
of Florida. Most of my colleagues never knew I'd had cancer.
They didn't know the things I'd been called, a "bone" when I was
a bone marrow transplant patient, or a "train wreck" when I went
septic. That I'd ever had "the killing crab," one resident's words
for cancer.

Along the way, I've heard the phrases for patients. Words used
to describe specific problems, like "squash rot" for brain deterioration, "sludge fest" for a patient with bowel problems, and "eaten
up" for a patient with metastasis. Words for places — "spit pit" and
"raw bar" for burn unit; "death traps" for surgical intensive care or
the bone marrow transplant unit, and "land of the five C's" for a
service filled with patients with diseases beginning with C, like
COPD (Chronic Obstructive Pulmonary Disease), CRI (Chronic
Renal Insufficiency), CHF (Congestive Heart Failure), craziness,
or cancer. There are words for mental status, like "Gorked" for
medicated beyond consciousness, or the "O" sign for patients
with wide-open mouths, and the "Q" sign for patients showing a
wide-open mouth and a protruding tongue.

But in all of medicine there are more phrases for dying than
anything else. "Crump," "Circle the drain," "Slow code," and
"Vegetable." There are hostile phrases like "FUBAR," or Fucked
Up Beyond Any Repair. And abbreviations — "RFB," or Ready for
Box, and "MFB," Measure for Box. Some of them have a hint of
humor, like "D/C to Maker," or discharge patient from hospital to
God, or "pickled" for an alcoholic, but most, like "crash," have a
hint of hostility.

Before I met the young surgeon, those phrases enraged me. I
felt the quick burn in my face when physicians distanced

themselves from me, calling me a bone or a train wreck. I was desperate that they see themselves in me, recognize my raw human terror in themselves. Drop the distance, reach across it, and offer comfort instead.

But after working with medical students and residents, I've come to understand that they do see themselves in me. These words are nothing more than a barometer of how primitively they cope. A measure of how little they've been taught about healthier ways to survive the horrible things they see every day. They use these words, these callused phrases, because they're the most available weapons they have, to flail and struggle against the realization that eventually we all die and then get measured for a box.

Otter Bar River Wisdom

The moment of truth has arrived. Our first rapids are coming. I look at the others. Jay's eyebrows are high on his head — *What have we gotten ourselves into?* — and Eric mouths the word "Wow." Chuck is white as a ghost but shrugs. This is my first vacation from my new job and now I'm starting to regret my suggestion that we all meet at a kayak school. We are at the Otter Bar Kayak School in Northern California, where the Klamath and Salmon Rivers run hard and fast in the early summer.

I'm wedged in a yellow Corsican whitewater kayak, my spray skirt tight around my middle, my knees and hips and feet tight in the small plastic boat. I'm in clear emerald green water and bubbles rise like silver coins around my bow. But we are floating toward a terrible roar. I swallow and tighten the grip on my paddle, vigilantly scanning the water near my bow. Nothing yet. My kayak instructor is yelling at me over the sound. I can't quite hear him. *Is he telling me to close my eyes? What?*

Reg Lake, a legend among kayakers, has long gray hair and a face blown smooth. In the 1970s Reg did many of the first descents of wild rivers in both the Northern and the Southern Hemispheres. He's told me stories of hiking fifteen miles into the mountains, a kayak strapped to his back, so he could be the first to surf and roll his way down foamy rapids that would later be named things like "Widow Maker" and "Churning Poison." Now he holds his paddle in one hand and cups his mouth with the other. "Close your eyes!" he insists.

"You're on drugs," I yell back, over the sound.

All day he has been trying to teach me to find the speed of the river. If I travel at the speed of the river, and don't fight it, it will take care of me, he says. It has the ring of pop psychology crap to me, but I'm learning that the river seems to agree with him.

He paddles toward me and I pretend not to notice him. He grabs my bow loop and pulls close. Now I can see the veins in his cheeks like purple firework traces. He repeats himself. I strain my neck to look down the river toward a rock outcropping where the water shoots around it, leaving a frothy wake, but I have to twist past his eyes to see and it feels rude not to look at him while he's talking, so I do. My kayak bobs for a moment, the water gathering steam before it shoots this way and that. I grow nervous and try to calm myself. I know if I flip here he will fish me out. He's already done it twice today.

"If I fill your kayak with rocks and send it down these rapids it'll show at the other end right side up. I promise."

I squint at him.

"I promise," he repeats. "Close your eyes."

So I trust him with his thick forearms and the sure way he holds his paddle, and taking a deep breath, I nervously seal my eyes. He lets go of my boat and I can sense the heart of the rapids coming from the intense sound. The kayak starts to bob and a spray of water hits my face. *Keep 'em shut, keep 'em shut, keep 'em shut.* I try to relax my shoulders and belly, but the sound is consuming and I can feel my boat spinning and bobbing. I remind myself to breathe. Gradually the sound eases and I open my eyes. I'm drifting backward, much slower than I expected, through relatively calm water. The roar I heard is not much more than a gurgle from here.

Relief! *Hey! I'm right side up!*

A heady proud feeling takes over. My first real rapids!

As part of my job I work with cancer patients referred from the University of Arizona Cancer Center. My patients come in for a variety of reasons, but the most common are folks facing their first treatments. When I meet an anxious chemotherapy first-timer, legs tapping, eyes vigilant, I borrow from Reg Lake. I grab him by the bow loop and ask him to close his eyes. I ask him to find the speed of the river and just ride it out. "You won't capsize," I assure him. "Open your mind to the possibility that you'll arrive safely downstream. There might be foam on your edges and a terrifying sound that eclipses every thought, but you won't capsize. Ride her out. Just ride her out."

Blindfolded

Dr. Frauenthal stands in the middle of the room. She trembles a little. The blindfold is tied behind her head and her hair flows over and around it. She tentatively lifts a leg high, higher than necessary, and takes a step. Her hands are out in front of her, open, with each finger reaching in a different direction. She bites her lip and makes a little sound as she steps. She's walking on a carpeted soft floor and she has nothing to fear, but each movement is tentative. A few more steps and she'll arrive in the arms of a colleague. She takes another timid step. And another. She is a hair away and then there. She exhales hard as the other's hands welcome her. She pulls off the blindfold and smiles.

I work in two departments at the University of Arizona, Psychiatry and Integrative Medicine. The Department of Integrative Medicine was started by Andy Weil, a national icon of sorts. I wear a number of hats in the program, but my fundamental role is to work with physicians, helping them unlearn years of denying their own needs, repressing their feelings about their patients, and not taking care of themselves. These days I give quite a few talks to health professionals around the country. With larger groups I perform my essays and chat a bit. With smaller groups I create experiences to communicate that to be a good doctor one must appreciate one's own humanity.

Twice a year I do a talk at Canyon Ranch, an upscale health spa in the eastern foothills of the Catalina Mountains here in Tucson. Physicians from all over the country attend these one-week programs. I usually get them for a few hours during one of the evenings. As part of the experience I ask them to join me in standing in a circle, facing inward. I ask for total silence. I blindfold one of them and ask him or her to stand in the middle. I spin them around and then gently send them walking toward the outskirts of the circle. When they reach the edge of the circle, they're stopped firmly by colleagues and sent back into the middle. They cross the circle a few times, blind, until I ask them to stop and take the blindfold off. It's harder than it sounds.

Inevitably they throw their hands up to guard themselves, or walk as if they are traveling through thick sand, feet lifted high. Some of them tilt their heads back, as if to ward off an attack from some lunging beast in their imaginations. Still others slow to a creeping walk, one tiny step in front of the next. In every group at least one of them stops cold, in the middle, too afraid to move. Eventually, with a little encouragement, they start again, one tentative step and another. Almost all of them smile in relief when they remove the blindfold.

Physicians aren't used to vulnerability; it's not part of their language, their understanding. They talk about procedures — spinal taps and bone marrow aspirations, biopsies and chemotherapy regimens — as if they were nothing more than having cable hooked up, or having a garbage disposal replaced. They are oblivious to what it feels like to wait, sleepless, in the darkest part of the morning, for surgery, a chemotherapy hit, a radiation treatment. They've been acculturated to ignore their own vulnerability, their own fears and hungers.

So I share it with them through this gentle exercise. A few simple steps in the dark, in the hopes that the next time they see one of us coming, they'll pause and offer comfort, help us see what they see, before sending us back across the dark circle alone.

En-trance

I didn't really want to go. An irrational fear. Like Terry's belief that if she watches the Indiana University Hoosiers play basketball, they'll lose. I still felt an increased vigilance in patient waiting rooms. The whispered greetings, schedule books and old magazines were unpleasantly familiar. Sitting there, appropriately coerced, I felt a restlessness, a pressure in my chest and arms. But I obliged and sat, dutifully trying to read a natural-health magazine.

Back in a patient exam room, Terry hopped up on the crinkly paper and smiled at me. I mocked, "Hey, that's my spot," and she giggled. I sat in the "family member chair" and spun around a few times. I studied the two framed posters, a quit-smoking poster of a duck with a cigarette in its mouth and a landscape print of a windmill. I ignored the large white machine next to Terry. We waited quietly.

Lynn Goolsby, our new doctor, knocked softly, entered, and approached Terry. She put a hand quickly on Terry's arm, a gentle greeting. They exchanged pleasantries. Lynn said a "hi" to me as she turned on the ultrasound machine.

I closed my eyes. *What horrible news will we get now?* I struggled to stay focused, swallowed, like before an exam. Terry reclined, her face toward the machine. Lynn spun some dials and moved something along Terry's belly. I heard a quick electric thumping. A rhythmic Morse code. Loud. *Is that an alarm?* "What is that?" I asked. On the screen I saw a tiny balloon inflating and deflating.

"Your baby's heartbeat." Lynn smiled. "It's strong."

For many months I avoided thinking about it. Even after the first kicks were reported to me, even after the little being waved at me through the ultrasound machine. I sifted each of Lynn's words for a sign of impending disaster. I waited for her to lean forward and explain what preeclampsia does, or gestational diabetes, or why Terry's alpha-fetoprotein tests signaled impending disaster. But Lynn just kept saying that everything looked good. She cooed and fawned over the black-and-white ultrasound photographs. "She's going to be beautiful," she said.

My parents visited when Terry was eight months pregnant. Reluc-
tantly, I went with Terry and them to Little Things, the store for
expectant mothers, to pick out a crib and changing bureau. The
salesgirl explained that we needed a theme for the baby's room—
Winnie the Pooh, or Noah's Ark, or Mickey and friends.

"Are we having a baby or putting on a play?" I asked.

Terry scowled at me and selected Noah's Ark. "We're going to
do this right," she said. She and my parents spent hours wandering the aisles, my mother carrying a copy of *Consumer Reports* with
pictures of car seats and bottles and portable cribs and diaper-
disposal vaults. My father pushed a cart behind her, making quiet
suggestions and occasionally shaking a selected item to test its
sturdiness. They smiled and hugged me more frequently than
usual, but still I resisted. I knew we were in the start of the fourth
act of *Hamlet* when things are looking up for a few minutes, before
Laertes and Ophelia and Hamlet die.

At Lamaze they showed us a movie of three couples. The first
couple looked like a professional birthing couple. He was clean-
shaven, nurturing, and had a smooth, breathy voice that could
have been on a hypnosis tape. He was never more than a few feet
from her, always touching her hair or stroking an arm, reminding
her to breathe and focus on him. She gave birth in only two
hours. The next couple showed what might happen if the baby
needed a C-section delivery. It showed how nervous they were
and then how everything turned out all right. The last couple was
from Boston. It showed the mom nine hours into labor, standing
in a shower. First she yelled at him, "Stop touching me!" and
slapped his hand away from her. He looked at the camera and
shrugged. Then she said to him, "I'm wicked nauseous." And he
responded, "Maybe you shouldn't have had that Philly cheese-
steak on the way to the hospital, eh?"

We all laughed. I felt relieved. If they could give birth, we could, too.

Then they showed the actual deliveries. It was amazing. Beautiful. Vaginas opening up like flowers to release beautiful little creatures. I cried and held Terry's arm. I looked around the room. All the men were crying and snuggling in next to the women. Then I noticed the women. They looked terrified. One of them said, "That's it. I'm not giving birth. This is over." She stood up. Her husband whispered something to her and she said, "Forget it. If you're so excited about it, *you* give birth to it."

The baby, of course, wouldn't come. We tried every old wives' trick we had ever heard of. We drove over bouncy roads, toasted with castor oil, had sex, took baths, and went for walks. Eventually Lynn decided to help the process along. The night before the planned event, Terry got a tape recorder and spoke into it about what she hoped for. When she turned the microphone toward me I studied my feet and whispered that I hoped the baby would be healthy. Terry nudged me and I fabricated some hopes about attending Vassar and having a sense of humor.

They gave us a great room. Windows overlooking Tucson. From her bed Terry could see the Catalina Mountains, Pusch Ridge and Finger Rock. She labored without medications and didn't complain. We played music and I tried to keep her occupied. Every time the monitoring machine whirred or beeped or hummed, I asked what it was. Has the disaster started? But Lynn was as soothing as ever, calmly announcing the progress in dilation centimeters and explaining to me, over and over, that the monitoring belt had slipped or shifted and everything was fine.

"Time to push," Lynn said finally.

When Terry opened and the little head peeked through I felt like I was standing on a wooden bridge over a crevasse. Wind and rain and life descending on me.

The small person Lynn pulled out of Terry was blue.

No.

Our nurse, smiling and joking a moment ago, leaned, serious, on an intercom button and calmly, too calmly, called for the Neonatal ICU team. "STAT," she said. A flock of sneakered feet poured into the room and whisked the blue being onto a warming table. I saw a tech squeezing a blue bag near her head.

"They're breathing for her," Lynn explained. "Stay calm. . . ."

No.

As if my elevator had snapped its cables, I felt the floor dropping; my heart thumped mercilessly. I noticed Terry's hand was wrapped in mine. She said something, but I was already adrift. Back there, in a carpeted room overlooking Gainesville. Watching my physician's thick fist pressed into his chin as he tried to explain the physiology of relapse, but his voice wouldn't come, the only sound from his mouth was the gasp of the bag inflating.

NO.

Then I was suddenly back in the room. Over the beeps and controlled voices, there was a loud trumpet call, brassy, filled with the music of urgent pleading. *A cry?* A proud, strong cry. And a pink little person was lifted, then settled like she'd done it a thousand times into her mother's arms. Eyes blinking. Feet wiggling. I heard a chorus of coos and "Ah there's," and Lynn said, "She's beautiful," and I knew Terry was smiling at me — but I couldn't take my eyes off Alexandra's tiny nails, on her tiny fingers, stretched, squeezing with life and endurance, around my thumb.

Dictated Chart Note

3/12/96

After a nine hour labor the patient gave birth to a healthy, 40 week gestation, female. Baby weighed 6 lbs. 13.4 oz. and was 19 inches long. By all parameters mother and baby appear healthy. Family thriving.

LYNN GOOLSBY, M.D.
University of Arizona Health Sciences Center

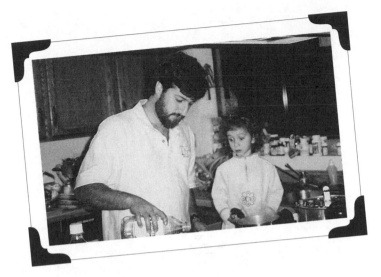

Part Seven

Learnings

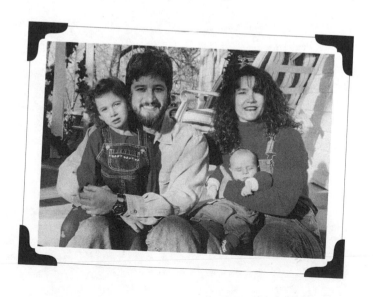

Mantra

Sometimes, when I'm about to do something nerve-racking, I recite them. The names of the chemotherapy drugs I took. The hard ones. I whisper them, alphabetically, to myself, as fast as I can so the words blend together. Before I asked my boss for a raise, before I told a colleague I didn't want to work with him anymore, before I watched the ultrasound machine for a heartbeat. While I recite them I can feel my shoulders dropping, my jaw unclenching, my fingers opening. "Adriamycin, bleomycin, Cytoxan, DTIC, nitrogen mustard, prednisone, procarbazine, vincristine, vinblastine, and VP-16."

My Kind of Garage Salesman

I was on the way back from a bagel run, obligatory in our house on Saturday morning, when I passed a hand-scratched sign: GARAGE SALE. I had to stop. I parked the car and started up the long drive. From the bottom of the drive I could see odds and ends scattered across tables—old ledgers and tablecloths, records and baskets. An older man sat in a metal chair watching a few shoppers. I love a good garage sale.

Before I got sick I could run into a large department store, get what I needed, and leave, having never looked at anyone. I remember going to return a watch, only to be embarrassed when I realized I didn't know who'd waited on me. I'd never looked at her.

When I was in treatment I was often dependent for social contact on the people around me. I needed them to see me as more than a cancer patient and I wanted to see them as more than interchangeable technicians. I started joking about bad-hair days with the woman who pushed my wheelchair and ten things to do with an I.V. pole on a Saturday night with the doc on call. I'd comment on a lapel pin worn by a cleaning woman or a technician's tattoo.

I never stopped. I still need to see the person behind the counter as more than a salesgirl, and I want them to see me, too. Before I rent it I need to discuss *Truly Madly Deeply* with the owner at Director's Chair Video, and Barbara Kingsolver's latest book with the information volunteer at Bookman's used bookstore, and the implications of having a daughter born in the Year of the Cat with Vy, my Vietnamese barber. Along the way I might share a few observations, like how I recently tried to pay for a meal with my bagel count card, or how maybe Ray's Market should give up the fancy computer register and go back to an abacus and beads. When I'm lucky I run into a shopkeeper with a bit of grit or humor, and maybe we spend a few extra minutes chatting.

I may unintentionally annoy other shoppers by talking so much with sales folk. I know I'm inefficient. I might even be a drag on the economy, slowing the rate of purchases. I don't want to bother anyone, but I'm also not willing to go back to how I was before. A large percentage of my life is made up of these small encounters, moments when two people can act human to each other, and I don't want to waste the opportunity anymore, assembly-line purchasing be damned.

———

When I got to the top of the drive at the garage sale, I got a closer look at the older man. His face had long lines running across it like an apricot pit. He looked to be in his eighties, sitting on a thin metal chair sewing a denim patch onto a flannel jacket. He looked up at me and then yelled toward the house with a weathered voice that carried: "Hey, Maggie! This one wants to buy something." Maggie responded from inside the house that she would be right out. "No rush," the older man called. "He hasn't found it yet," and he winked at me.

This could take a while.

Phosphorescence

the persistent emission of light without burning
or appreciable heat

When I was sixteen I was in love with Amy, a beautiful, creative girl who loved me back for a summer when we were at Camp Woodstock, a YMCA camp in northern Connecticut. My memories of her are mingled with bug juice, swamped canoes, and campfire smoke. After camp we visited a fellow camper who lived on the beach in Rhode Island. While our friend argued with her parents about her college plans, we took a barefooted walk together out on the beach. It was cloudy, moonless, and there was barely enough light to see the sand dollars and crabs. When we got down near the water I felt my heart jump: In the surf we could see electric green swaths of light, like falling stars. As we got closer the green light was brighter. We stood at the edge of the water, wordless. When I looked down I saw that where our legs touched the water there were little twinkling speckles of green.

Amy smiled and stripped off her sweatshirt, bra, and shorts. "Come on," she beckoned, and dove into the cold water. Every slight move she made with her hands, breasts, and legs left a wake of bright green traces, and she glowed, surrounded by the light. I pulled off my T-shirt and shorts and followed her into the brisk water, watching the magic around my hands and feet. When I dove under I was bathed in the glow, and I felt a lightness in my chest. We pressed together, shivering and giggling, her face radiant.

These days, at the medical school, I spend much of my time around scientists. They are disciples of statistics and math, hypotheses and probability. They thrive on certainty. A right way to do things, a wrong way. They'd tell me that I owe my life to high-dose chemotherapy and radiation — and I'd agree. But sometimes I play with the idea that survival was due to something else, something more magical. Because between the cracks and fissures of science, there are still moments, seventeen years later, when I feel myself bathed in a magical green light that I can't and don't want to explain.

Body Bonus

Before chemotherapy I didn't know my veins. I wasn't in touch with the highways, thoroughfares, and back streets of my hands and arms. I couldn't read a vein's chemotherapy age from its color and thickness. I had no experience with hardened bicycle brake cables, had no favorite paths or loved intersections. But now I know them. Each turn of the antecubital, the dorsum. And I feel the life inside them. My pulse. I feel it when grabbing a steering wheel, writing a chart note, or even resting my hand in my lap. It's a grounding sensation. It says, "This is where you are right now, this is what your body thinks." Sometimes, when I pull my car into the driveway to find Terry's old Toyota already there, I feel a pleasant quickening, the slightly faster beat, the metronome of my life turned up just one notch. *Thump thump. Thump thump.*

And I know other things now. I know that I chew the inside of my right cheek when I'm stressed. Now when my tongue finds that thin crease, a narrow line from the hinge of my jaw to the corner of my mouth, I know I've been packing too much kindling on the fire. I know that I eat when I feel afraid. That I'm capable of reaching for the popcorn popper with one hand while the other does its five-finger dance, hunting for tumors. That my stomach does not know the difference between tides of fear and pangs for food.

Before the weakness, too fragile to push open doors and climb stairs, I did not celebrate a stride. I would never have thought to throw my head back and sing after a lung-grabbing sprint.

Before chemotherapy I didn't smell the world. One strange outcome of a brain hunting for the source of poison is its willingness to invest more resources in olfaction. Now I automatically search the world for scents, both colorful and noxious. An old familiar perfume, the desert after it rains, mesquite burning — any smell can gather me up and spin me away.

I'm not glad to have had cancer. I'd trade the gift of living fully in my body for a chemotherapy-free lifetime. But I was never offered a trade, so I'll enjoy this. *Thump thump. Thump thump.*

Speed

I stopped and chatted with Jim, one of the guys I play Ultimate Frisbee with. We were on the losing team and had lost the field. We were sitting together on the ground and started talking. I enjoy talking with him; he's one of those rare guys who's willing to talk openly about work, children, and fatherhood. I love these conversations, when I can talk openly with another man the way women do so easily with one another. We started with money worries, how expensive day care is, and mortgage insurance, and then he moved us into more delicate waters. "You know, the thing that really bothers me is that Alice and I don't have sex much anymore 'cause we're both so tired. I haven't been to a movie in over a year, which used to be my favorite thing, and I can't remember the last time I had a complete night's sleep." I nodded and then listed my gripes, mostly about grant applications and too many patients to care for with too little time, and then I described a yelling match I'd had with Alexandra about what she'd wear to day care, and we nodded in silence for a minute.

"But being a dad," he suggested, "is still the best thing ever, huh?" I agreed and we moved into the obligatory bragging phase of the conversation. He told me how his daughter turns into his shadow the minute he gets home and how he looks forward to her hug all day. I told him about Alex's giggling. Then we escalated. I reported that Alexandra, now three, had recently set up a chessboard without assistance. His little girl, the same age, had managed to videotape her favorite show. We crowed for a while longer and then he scratched his arm and looked down.

"You know," he said, softer, "I can't tell where the time went. It goes so fast. Jessica was just born yesterday, but now she's three.

The time shoots by. I spend more time with her than most of my friends spend with their kids, but I still feel like I'm missing everything. Not just time with her, but my whole life, just shooting by."

I thought about what he said right then, and again later that night and the next day. I remembered how time changed on chemotherapy. Kneeling on the linoleum for minutes that felt like hours, the infusions and the tin taste in my mouth that lingered as time slowed to a crawl. Then I realized that for me, a sense that time is spinning along quickly is comforting. It isn't the portent of a missed life but the badge of an enjoyed one. When agony visited me, life didn't get less busy, it just turned slow. Painfully slow. My experience of time doesn't have anything to do with busyness or attention, it has to do with enjoyment and fullness.

I love this speed, my life breezing by as if I were standing in a convertible, autumn sunshine bathing my cheeks, shoulders and open hands.

Nana's Legacy

Nana is now ninety years old. She wears purple jogging sneakers and *Risky Business* sunglasses when she's in the sun. She goes to Gym and Swim at the Jewish Community Center five days a week. She bobs in the water and swims and does calisthenics. She visits with friends and gossips. On the weekends she sells fashion cards she makes from scraps of fabric and she practices piano. At night she listens to her operas on the tapes her daughter made for her.

There is an enlarged photograph of Nana in my office. She's standing, torso deep, in an Olympic pool. Her arms are raised

high and her head is tossed back. The waves around her create a
confluence of shadow and glitter. In her face I can see the smile of
a much younger girl. Her eyes are confident and her palms are
open, facing the camera. Her face says, *I am unconquerable.*

We speak a couple times a month by phone. When I ask her
how she's doing she says, "Not enough hours in the day," her voice
melodic, pronunciations tickled with German. "I'm a happy old
woman," she tells me. In her voice there's no trace of her history.
Of the family she lost to the Gestapo, the Coventry bombings that
left her standing in her kitchen, looking into the night sky where
the ceiling used to be, or the three times she lost everything but
the things she could carry. There's no sign of the anguish from
burying a husband, fifty years ago, in a grassy pasture on another
continent, or the struggle of raising two headstrong children
alone, in a country where she didn't speak the language.

Her hands show it. They're thick and curled from labor, scrub-
bing pots and bathtubs. And her back, broad and hunched. But
more than anything, the random possessions around her apartment
show it. Nana still saves things. I learned this when my mother and I
helped her move to a smaller place. My surprise started in her bathroom. Next to her tub I found a stack of junk mail. There were old
stickers from magazine contests, coupons for marmalade, and
credit-card offers with great introductory rates. In a closet I found
empty mayonnaise and peanut butter jars, washed and stacked, lids
like fallen dominos in a long row. Under her piano I found used
business envelopes, pressed flat, tied with string and stored neatly.
Near the wall I found an old coffee can, *good to the last drop,* filled
with Avon sampler lipsticks.

As I carried boxes through the small apartment, which I'd visited hundreds of times, I noticed things I'd never seen before. Her
candle holders are shampoo bottle caps. Her window shade drawstrings are paper clips covered with lace. The glasses she serves
lemonade in are jelly jars. And each saved shoe, each coupon,

each paper clip—each is a musical note in a symphony of resilience. A resounding reminder that all lives are visited by crises. That with creativity and a willingness to forge small solutions, a shampoo cap here, a patch of fabric there, we endure.

Bedrock

Alexandra likes popcorn. Like me. She likes pizza. Like me. She likes staying up late watching movies. She likes water, laying her head back until her ears are submerged, looking up at the clouds. She likes lightning. She likes bare feet. She likes to sing into the bathroom mirror. She likes big towels and little orange wedges. She likes to pet our cats' bellies more than their heads. She gets irritable and irrational when she's hungry. She gets restless after she eats, she needs to move. She gets snippy when she's tired. She likes to hang upside down whenever she can. She likes to wait for me behind a door, growling suddenly and then giggling at my surprise. She likes to sleep in small spaces, curled up tight against the things she loves. Like me.

She has the same curve in her cheek, the same hands, and exactly the same eyes. Green and yellow and brown. Terry likes to look into Alex and tell her she got her daddy's face and eyes and laugh.

I know that Alex wouldn't be here if my mother hadn't had a conversation with a stranger. It's hard to reconcile that knowledge with how permanent she seems when she's slurping blueberries, or asking if she can have Fritos for breakfast, or painting my toenails hot pink, her face opened in a wide grin. It feels as if she's always been here. But at other times, like when her little belly rises and falls and she snores a little, and I sit in her bedroom to watch her because I can't find any other passage to sleep, at those moments I can feel the thin thread that led her here. When the house is still and time slows. And then the fragility of her life and mine rises in me like hot mercury.

It wasn't until I fell in love with her—real love, with its bone-gnawing vulnerability and irrepressible tingle—that what my mother did made sense. It's as if a curtain opened when she was born, revealing a stage filled with new feelings. Like the peaceful willingness to strip this life off if she needed it. A hunger to watch her when she doesn't know I'm there. And sometimes a new weariness when it's nearing my bedtime and she's still singing her rendition of "Rockin' Robin," with emphasis on the "Tweet tweet tweet."

But now, twelve years later, I get it. How, only eight hours after our heated exchange, my antidrug-never-apologize mom could plant a weed she despised in our backyard. How she could sacrifice fundamental beliefs in favor of her child's comfort. Now I understand that down there, below all of my beliefs, even the ones I thought I'd forged in steel and concrete, there's bedrock more solid than anything built atop it.

As I write these words Alex is wearing a purple costume with a cape and a wand. She prances through my study. She tells me, matter-of-fact, that she's the king and the queen and the fair maiden. When I ask her if she's the entire kingdom she nods. "Sure, I think so."

And I guess I think so too.

Dictated Chart Note: Radiology

11/1/99

This is a 34-year-old married white male with a remote history of Hodgkin's Disease who presents for evaluation. X-Ray and CT Scan show no evidence of disease. Mediastinal and side views clear.

JAKE ENDE, M.D.
University of Arizona College of Medicine

Mom's Marijuana: Part D

Dad wanted to do it in September, after I left for graduate school. Southern New England cooled for a few days in early September, teasing the sweltering population, and then gave one last humid blast. The temperature even climbed into the hundreds. They turned on the big fan, built into the attic floor. The stench filled the house. He told her he felt strongly about it, let's do it! But Mom silenced him.

"Not yet. You never know," she said.

My parents take the winter coats into the attic after the season's last gasp. It's usually signaled by the first purple crocus peeking up between the wood chips in the front yard and the tree frogs starting their evening chorus. Dad said he saw it all up there. Draped over the beams. The smell still strong. "Do we really want all of our coats to smell of this?" he asked her.

"Not yet. You never know," she said.

In November, when he took the coats down, we learned he was right. Everything smelled, including his favorite black overcoat, the one with the thin lapels, as well as his Greek fisherman's cap and the gloves Grandma knitted him with the zigzag lines and the huge thumb. Dad said he found Mom in the kitchen, her face buried in the Sunday crossword, and offered his overcoat as evidence.

"Here, smell this!" he insisted.

"Not yet. You never know," she said.

It was still up there when he brought down the menorah a few months later. And then when he put it back. And when he went to find the South American bird book for their trip to Guatemala in May. And when the bike rack wasn't in the garage in August. And when he couldn't find the photograph of Grandma when she was eleven, all teeth and frills, to blow up for her eightieth birthday in March. And season after season.

"Not yet. You never know."

One morning last winter Mom appeared in Dad's study wearing coveralls and gloves. "What would you say to cleaning out the attic?" she asked him.

"You mean?" he perked.

"Yup," she said, and handed him a lawn bag.

They climbed the steep stairs and filled the bags with the old curled leaves, stiff branches, and dried buds. Dad carried the vacuum up the steps and sucked up what was left. He even moved the box of old books in the corner so he could vacuum behind it.

Then they dragged the bags into the backyard, to the bare plot of land they use as a garden. Mom put some crumpled newspaper down in the middle of the cold soil and Dad emptied the dry mass on top, ten pounds of old marijuana leaves and branches. She leaned over and struck a match. When it was lit they stood back, away from the smoke, and watched. Mom said it burned fast, branches crackling and smoke rising into the cool morning air.

This April we visited. When I was carrying our bags into the house, I noticed the white-snow bunting crocuses were fully opened, bright orange blooms inside. Sparrows and finches surrounded the feeders hanging in the sycamore and I could smell freshly cut grass.

The next morning Terry and I awoke late, still on western time. When I checked David's old room Alexandra's bed was empty and her sneakers were gone. Already up. I wandered out onto the porch in my shorts and sweatshirt. From there I could see Mom and Alex. They were in the garden.

Mom was kneeling, talking softly with Alex, who held a small plant in her hands. Mom scooped out some soil and Alex carefully placed the plant in the ground. They covered it over and Mom pushed a small stake in the ground next to it. Then Alex lifted a tall container of water. Mom tried to help her, but Alex said, "I want to do it!" and Mom let her drip a few drops over the plant. They moved a foot or so and did it again. After a while Mom said something and Alex looked up at me and waved, exuberant. "I'm planting! I'm planting!" she yelled.

"You're planting tomatoes!" Mom said to Alex.

"They'll be huge," Alex said up to me, holding her hands as wide as they could go. "Big tomatoes."

"We'll mail you all of the results," Mom called up to me.

"That's okay. Really. Torture your neighbors." Alex picked up another plant. "Come on, Bubbie!" she implored. But Mom was still looking at me.

"She's good at this, it's in her blood," Mom said.

Then she turned, kneeled next to my daughter, and helped her put the small plant in the ground.

Epilogue

I'm sitting here in Tucson, Arizona, at one of my favorite spots in the world. I'm behind my desk, looking up into the Santa Catalina mountains out the window of my study. It's been terrific to write this book and I've already started to mourn its completion. So much so that I've been thinking of ways to keep it going, like sending notes in to torture Shaye, my editor. Adding paragraphs here, taking some away there. I could probably continue forever if I didn't think Shaye would change her phone number.

Terry is back working in the bone marrow transplant unit here where she regularly saves lives and I've started doing talks around the country, mostly to health professionals. I still enjoy seeing patients and writing at the University of Arizona, but more than anything I like chasing my daughters around. We are healthy and happy. Scans are clear.

Since the final version of the book was written, our lives have changed in an important way. We've welcomed Abigail Ilse into our family, a beautiful girl and another product of the sperm saved in 1987. This means I am now surrounded by three women. Stay tuned for the sequel to this book, entitled *House of Estrogen.*

I am the luckiest man I know.

DAN SHAPIRO, SPRING 2000